Essenti[...]

of PSYCHOLOGIC[...]

Everything you need to know to administer, interpret, and score the major psychological tests.

Essentials of Psychological Assessment Series

Series Editors, Alan S. Kaufman and Nadeen L. Kaufman

Essentials of WAIS-III Assessment
by Alan S. Kaufman and Elizabeth O. Lichtenberger

Essentials of Millon Inventories Assessment
by Stephen N. Strack

Essentials of CAS Assessment
by Jack A. Naglieri

Essentials of Forensic Psychological Assessment
by Marc J. Ackerman

Essentials of Bayley Scales of Infant Development–II Assessment
by Maureen M. Black and Kathleen Matula

Essentials of Myers-Briggs Type Indicator® Assessment
by Naomi Quenk

Essentials of WISC-III and WPPSI-R Assessment
by Alan S. Kaufman and Elizabeth O. Lichtenberger

Essentials of Rorschach Assessment
by Tara Rose, Michael Maloney, and Nancy Kaser-Boyd

Essentials of Career Interest Assessment
by Jeff Prince and Lisa J. Heiser

Essentials of Cross-Battery Assessment
by Dawn P. Flanagan and Samuel O. Ortiz

Essentials of Cognitive Assessment with KAIT and Other Kaufman Measures
by Elizabeth O. Lichtenberger, Debra Broadbooks, and Alan S. Kaufman

Essentials

of Nonverbal Assessment

R. Steve McCallum

Bruce A. Bracken

John D. Wasserman

John Wiley & Sons, Inc.
NEW YORK · CHICHESTER · WEINHEIM · BRISBANE · SINGAPORE · TORONTO

Library of Congress Cataloging-in-Publication Data:
McCallum, R. Steve.
    Essentials of nonverbal assessment / Steve McCallum, Bruce Bracken, John Wasserman.
        p. cm. — (Essentials of psychological assessment series)
    Includes bibliographical references (p. 236) and index.
    ISBN 0-471-38318-X (pbk. : alk. paper)
        1. Intelligence tests for preliterates.   I. Bracken, Bruce A.   II. Wasserman, John
(John D.)   III. Title.   IV. Series.

    BF432.5.I55   M33   2000
    153.9'334—dc21

                                                                        00-042268

Printed in the United States of America.
10 9 8 7 6 5 4 3 2 1

To my students.
—RSM

To everyone who has been influential in my life—family, friends, colleagues, and students—and with special love to Mary Jo and Bruce Jr.
—BAB

To my mother, who is an expert in nonverbal communication.
—JDW

CONTENTS

SERIES PREFACE

I n the *Essentials of Psychological Assessment* series, our goal is to provide the reader with books that deliver key practical information in the most efficient and accessible style. The series features instruments in a variety of domains, such as cognition, personality, education, and neuropsychology. For the experienced clinician, books in the series offer a concise, yet thorough, way to master the continuously evolving supply of new and revised instruments, as well as a convenient method for keeping up to date on the tried-and-true measures. The novice will find here a prioritized assembly of all the information and techniques that must be at one's fingertips to begin the complicated process of individual psychological diagnosis.

Wherever feasible, visual shortcuts to highlight key points are utilized alongside systematic, step-by-step guidelines. Chapters are focused and succinct. Topics are targeted for an easy understanding of the essentials of administration, scoring, interpretation, and clinical application. Theory and research are continually woven into the fabric of each book, but always to enhance clinical inference, never to sidetrack or overwhelm. We have long been advocates of "intelligent" testing—the notion that a profile of test scores is meaningless unless it is brought to life by the clinical observations and astute detective work of knowledgeable examiners. Test profiles must be used to make a difference in the child's or adult's life, or why bother to test? We want this series to help our readers become the best intelligent testers they can be.

The assessment of nonverbal intelligence has long been of paramount importance because this type of assessment permits the evaluation of diverse groups of individuals who might otherwise be assessed unfairly or not at all. The use of nonverbal intelligence tests has permitted fairer evaluation of the cognitive abilities of individuals with hearing impairments, autism, and other disorders of language; of those who are bilingual or do not speak English at all; and of those whose cultural differences render any kind of verbal test of questionable validity. In *Essentials of Nonverbal Assessment,* the authors provide readers with a thorough and insightful treatment of the most commonly used nonverbal tests available, both unidimensional and comprehensive. Their goal is to provide examiners with the array of information needed to competently assess and diagnose children who do not use English as their primary means of communication and for whom traditional language-loaded (and, typically, culture-saturated) tests would be inappropriate. This book will be quite useful for promoting fairer intellectual assessment of several key populations of children and adolescents.

Alan S. Kaufman, PhD, and Nadeen L. Kaufman, EdD, Series Editors
Yale University School of Medicine

One

OVERVIEW: ASSESSING DIVERSE POPULATIONS WITH NONVERBAL TESTS OF INTELLIGENCE

Recently, a number of nonverbal intelligence tests have been developed. These tests vary along several dimensions, including fairness, comprehensiveness, psychometric quality, representativeness of standardization, appropriateness for individuals versus groups, and so on. In this book we describe the best of these. Our goal is to provide an easy reference for users of these tests. Readers will find this book easy to read and to use. Directions are provided for administration, scoring, and interpretation for each test, as are descriptions of strengths and weaknesses. Important points are highlighted by Rapid Reference, Caution, and Don't Forget boxes. Each chapter contains a brief summary and a self-test to help you summarize and consolidate the content. The content should help you become competent in the use and clinical interpretation of nonverbal tests.

Essentials of Nonverbal Assessment is organized systematically. In Chapter One the reader will find a rationale for the use of nonverbal intelligence tests, a brief history of nonverbal assessment, a discussion of the distinction between unidimensional and multidimensional tests, and an introduction to individually administered tests. Finally, as in every chapter, there is a brief summary, followed by a self-test. Chapter Two provides an introduction to unidimensional tests and a description of the administration, scoring, strengths and weaknesses, and clinical application of six unidimensional tests: BETA III (Kellogg & Morton, 1999), the Comprehensive Test of Nonverbal Intelligence (CTONI; Hammill, Pearson, & Wiederholt, 1996), the General Ability Measure for Adults (GAMA; Naglieri & Bardos, 1997), the Naglieri Nonverbal Ability Test (NNAT; Naglieri, 1996), the Raven's Progressive Matrices (RPM; Raven, Raven, & Court, 1998), and the Test of Nonverbal Intelligence–Third Edition (TONI-III; Brown, Sherbenou, & Johnsen, 1997). Chapter Three introduces multidimensional tests in general and provides a detailed description of one such test, the Universal Nonverbal Intelligence Test (UNIT; Bracken & Mc-Callum, 1998). Directions for administration, scoring, and interpretation are provided, along with a description of clinical application strategies. Chapter Four presents a detailed description of UNIT's psychometric properties and clinical strengths and weaknesses, as well as a case study. Chapter Five provides directions for administration, scoring, and interpretation of the Leiter International Performance Scale–Revised (Leiter-R; Roid & Miller, 1997), as well as strategies for its clinical application. Finally, Chapter Six addresses specific strengths and weaknesses of the Leiter-R and presents a case study.

RATIONALE FOR AND HISTORY OF NONVERBAL INTELLECTUAL ASSESSMENT

Tests of cognitive and intellectual ability are valued because they are capable of predicting important academic and vocational outcomes (Bracken, 1993; Hunter & Hunter, 1984; Jensen, 1980). In addition, tests provide information considered useful by clinicians for diagnostic and intervention purposes (Kaufman, 1994). In the western world, productive efforts to assess intelligence began in the nineteenth century. From the beginning, test developers have faced the challenge of assessing the cognitive functioning of individuals who lack the ability to demonstrate their cognitive skills using the language of the culture in which they live. For example, during the early 1800s, French clinicians were among the first to propose and attempt methods to assess and remediate the intellectual abilities of children with limited language capabilities. In a famous early case, Jean Itard attempted to assess the cognitive abilities of the Wild Boy of Aveyron in an effort to determine whether the youth could acquire functional language skills (Carrey, 1995; Itard, 1932). Other historical figures have pursued the problem of assessing the intellectual abilities of children who could not or would not speak. Seguin (1907) is well known for his development of unique instrumentation to aid in the assessment of children's abilities through nonverbal means. Seguin's instrument required the placement of common, puzzle-like geometric shapes into inserts of the same shape. The instrument, known universally as the Seguin Form Board, has been modified and in various forms has become widely used internationally.

Not until the twentieth century did the press for nonverbal assessment become especially important in the United States. During World War I, the armed forces needed methods to assess the abilities of foreign-born and illiterate military recruits, in addition to the typical literate, English-speaking recruits. Consequently, the Committee on the Psychological Examination of Recruits was formed, and it included some of the most noted psychologists of the time (Thorndike & Lohman, 1990). According to the *Examiner's Guide for the Army Psychological Examination* (Government Printing Office, 1918), military testing was used to classify soldiers according to mental ability, create organizational units of equal strength, identify potential problem soldiers, assist in training and assignments, identify potential officers, and discover soldiers with special talents or skills. Ultimately, the Army Mental Tests resulted in both Alpha and Beta forms. The Group Examination Alpha (Army Alpha) was administered to recruits who could read and respond to the written English version of the scale. Because the Army Alpha was limited as a measure of ability when recruits had limited English proficiency or were illiterate, the Group Examination Beta portion of the Mental Tests (Army Beta) was developed as a nonverbal supplement to Army Alpha. In addition, the army also developed the Army Performance Scale Examination, an individually administered test for use with individuals who could not be tested effectively in group form using the Alpha and Beta tests. The Army Performance Scale Examination and the Army Beta served an important need, especially in a country with a population as diverse as that of the United States. They included a variety of performance tasks, many of which were to appear later on the Wechsler Scales (e.g., puzzles, cube constructions, digit symbols, mazes, picture completions, picture arrangements). Some of these included tasks pioneered by Kohs (1919), Seguin (1907), Porteus (1915), and Pintner and Patterson (1917).

Nonverbal tests were also developed in the private sector during this time. In 1924, G. Arthur took over the development of a test that ultimately became known as the Arthur Point Scale of Performance Tests (Arthur, 1943, 1947). The Point Scale was begun in 1917 under the guidance of Herbert Woodrow (Arthur, 1925; Arthur & Woodrow, 1919). Development of the Point Scale represents an important milestone because it combined and modified a variety of existing performance tests—including a revision of the Knox Cube Test (Knox, 1914), Seguin Form Board, Arthur Stencil Design Test, Porteus Maze Test (Porteus, 1915), and an adaptation of the Healy Picture Completion Test (Healy, 1914, 1918, 1921)—into a battery. The Point Scale was intended for individuals who were deaf or otherwise hard of hearing and who were therefore distinctly disadvantaged when administered language-loaded intelligence tests. Arthur's goal was to create a nonverbal battery that collectively would "furnish an IQ comparable to that obtained with the Binet scales" (Arthur, 1947, p. 1).

By the middle of the twentieth century, nonverbal tests were being used for a variety of purposes, well beyond assessment of cross-cultural or illiterate populations. For example, nonverbal procedures also were needed to assess the cognitive abilities of people with neurological impairments (e.g., traumatic brain injury), psychiatric conditions (e.g., selective/elective mutism, autism), speech and language disorders, and learning disabilities, as well as other language-related conditions. Essentially, nonverbal assessment procedures were needed for all individuals for whom traditional language-loaded intelligence tests had not provided an accurate representation of the individual's true current level of intellectual functioning. In this sense, nonverbal tests of intelligence were designed to reduce the bias associated with influences of language, that is, to remove the language confound associated with measuring intelligence. When general intelligence is the targeted construct, the heavy verbal demands of most language-loaded intelligence tests can create unfair construct-irrelevant" influences on the examinee's performance (Brown, Reynolds, & Whitaker, 1999; Hilliard, 1984; Reynolds, Lowe, & Saenz, 1999). Just as all group administered tests with written directions and content become primarily "reading tests" for individuals with poor reading skills, all tests with verbal direction and content become primarily "language tests" for individuals with limited language proficiency.

Efforts to develop "culture fair" tests over the past few decades have met with only limited success (e.g., R. B. Cattell's Culture Fair Intelligence Test). Despite authors' best efforts, it has not been possible to develop truly culture fair tests of ability (Frijda & Jahoda, 1966), in part because all tests are "anchored in an originating culture" (Lonner, 1985). Braden (1999) argued that rather than working toward the goal of developing measures of cognitive abilities that are independent of cultural diversity, researchers might better "disentangle the related constructs of cognitive ability and diversity" (p. 352) by seeking to create objective measures of diversity.

Some of the early nonverbal tests were adopted by psychologists and used extensively (e.g., Leiter International Performance Scale; Leiter, 1959, 1948; Columbia Mental Maturity Scale; Burgemeister, Blum, & Lorge, 1972; Draw a Person; Goodenough, 1926). However, these tests eventually fell into disfavor because their norms, stimulus materials, or procedures became outdated. The failure among test publishers to revise and renorm these few remaining nonverbal instruments created an even greater void in the nonverbal armament of practicing psychologists.

Consequently, many psychologists began to rely on tests with language-reduced "performance" tasks from standard batteries in an effort to provide fairer assessments. In this context, the Performance Scale of the Wechsler Intelligence Scale for Children (WISC; Wechsler, 1949) and its later editions became one of the most popular "nonverbal" tests, and was regularly used when children's hearing or language skills were considered a confound. Ironically, few psychologists seemed to notice or object that each of the Wechsler Performance subtests has test directions that are heavily laden with wordy verbal instructions and basic language concepts (Bracken, 1986; Kaufman, 1990, 1994).

The developing void in the availability of current nonverbal tests of ability and psychologists' growing recognition of the limitations associated with using language-reduced performance scales have resulted in a proliferation of nonverbal intelligence tests during the 1990s. It also is likely that increased social awareness and heightened sensitivity among psychologists has increased the acceptance of nonverbal assessment procedures. The demand for nonverbal assessment instrumentation and procedures is becoming increasingly strong because of the rapidly shifting world population and the influx of immigrants into communities of all sizes and in all regions throughout the United States.

Traditionally, immigrants have resettled in large metropolitan areas on the East and West coasts of the United States and psychologists who work in these coastal cities learned to anticipate that many languages would be spoken by the children in their urban schools. More recently, the immigrant resettlement efforts of many religious institutions and social organizations have encouraged more immigrants to settle in nontraditional regions and locales (e.g., midwestern regions, rural locations, southern gulf coastal areas). For example, Vietnamese immigrants have settled in large numbers along the Texas and Louisiana Gulf Coast, where they have become active in the shrimping industry. Similarly, Cubans and Hmong have resettled in colder, rural locations, such as Wisconsin and Minnesota. The result of such geographic dispersion among immigrant groups is that many communities that were once fairly homogeneous in race, ethnicity, culture, and language are now multicultural, multilingual, multiethnic, and multiracial.

Although cities have always been considered the center of this country's melting pot, the actual number of immigrants, the diverse nationalities represented, and the variety of languages spoken in our urban schools are truly staggering. For example, it has been reported that more than 200 languages are spoken by the children who attend the Chicago city schools (Pasko, 1994)! Moreover, Chicago is not unique. More than 1.4 million children who have limited English proficiency (LEP) are estimated to reside in California (Puente, 1998), with more than 140 languages represented in this population (Unz, 1997).

As might be expected, schools in the southwestern United States have large populations of English *and* Spanish speaking children. However, somewhat surprising is the very large number of other languages that are also spoken throughout this region of the country. For example, 67 languages are spoken by the students in the Tempe, Arizona school system (Ulik, 1997) and more than 50 languages are spoken in the nearby community school district of Scottsdale (Steele, 1998). Also in the southwest, the schools of Plano, Texas report that their student body collectively speaks more than 60 languages (Power, 1996). There has long been a need for Spanish-speaking bilingual psychologists and Spanish language tests throughout the southwest. However, there is also a less obvious yet equally important need for multilingual psychologists to competently serve the children who speak the scores of languages other than English and Spanish in this region.

Other regions of the country report similar levels of linguistic and cultural diversity among their student populations. For example, diverse student bodies are just as prevalent in the schools throughout the southeastern United States as in the southwest. Recent reports claim that in the southeast more than 80 languages are spoken in Palm Beach County Schools (Fast Fact, 1996); 54 languages are spoken in Broward County (Florida) schools (Donzelli, 1996); 48 languages are spoken in Prince William County, Virginia schools (O'Hanlon, 1997); and 45 languages are spoken by students in Cobb County, Georgia (Stepp, 1997). The list of communities with similarly diverse school populations grows ever longer, with a continually increasing number of languages spoken in urban and rural public schools throughout the country. Rapid Reference 1.1 shows many of the cities with large foreign-speaking populations in their schools.

≡Rapid Reference 1.1

Number of Languages Spoken in Various U.S. Public Schools

Chicago, IL:	200	(Pasko, 1994)
California:	140	(Unz, 1997)
Palm Beach, FL:	80	(Fast Fact, 1996)
Tempe, AZ:	67	(Ulik, 1997)
Plano, TX:	60	(Power, 1996)
Knoxville, TN:	61	(Forester, 2000)
Des Plaines, IL:	57	(Van Duch, 1997)
Broward County, FL:	54	(Donzelli, 1996)
Scottsdale, AZ:	50	(Steele, 1998)
Prince William, VA:	48	(O'Hanlon, 1997)
Cobb County, GA:	45	(Stepp, 1997)
Tukwila, WA:	30	(Searcey, 1998)
Schenectady, NY:	22	(Lipman, 1997)

Recently, some states have examined legislation that requires that children be assessed in their native language. Obviously such legislation presents problems for children and for the psychologists who are charged with assessing them. Although quality test translations are both possible and available (e.g., Bracken, 1998a; Bracken, Barona, Bauermeister, Howell, Poggioli, & Puente, 1990; Bracken & Fouad, 1987; Munoz-Sandoval, Cummins, Alvarado, & Ruef, 1998), test translations and subsequent norming and validation efforts are both costly and time consuming for a single dominant language (e.g., Spanish), let alone 200 or more low-incidence languages. Given the relative unavailability of quality translated tests and the very limited number of bilingual school psychologists, the primary alternative to testing children in their native languages is to remove language as a variable and employ nonverbal tests (Frisby, 1999). Rapid Reference 1.2 shows some of the difficulties associated with using translated tests.

Nonverbal tests of intelligence have been available for decades, but the 1990s have marked a resurgence in the development and improved quality of these

=Rapid Reference 1.2

··

**Some Problems Associated
with Using Translated Tests**

1. Translations are labor intensive
   and expensive
2. Translations require considerable
   time
3. Translations would be needed for
   every language spoken in an area
4. Translations cannot represent all
   the subtle but important regional
   differences within a language
5. There is a lack of skilled bilingual
   translators
6. There is a lack of skilled bilingual
   examiners

instruments. Psychologists currently have several nonverbal tests of intelligence from which to choose, depending on their individual needs and the nature of their referrals. With increased professional interest in nonverbal assessment and nonverbal instrumentation has come a concomitant refinement of knowledge, procedures, and practices. This growing field has also experienced some necessary refinement in terminology.

Because the terms "nonverbal assessment" and "nonverbal intellectual assessment" have often been used loosely, and frequently connote different meanings, these terms warrant definition. Bracken and McCallum (1998) use the term "nonverbal assessment" to describe a test administration process in which no receptive or expressive language demands are placed on *either* the examinee or the examiner. That is, during a nonverbal test administration there should be no spoken test directions and there should be no spoken responses required of the examinee. Many test manuals for extant "nonverbal tests" claim that the tests are administered in a nonverbal manner, but most of these tests are administered with verbal directions. Most "nonverbal tests," in fact, are best described as language-reduced instruments with verbal directions—sometimes with lengthy and complex verbal directions. For example, the Wechsler Performance Scale, and the Nonverbal Scales of the Kaufman Assessment Battery for Children (K-ABC; Kaufman & Kaufman, 1983), and the Differential Ability Scales (DAS; Elliott, 1990) are all presented with verbal directions. Each of these "nonverbal scales" requires that examinees understand spoken test directions before they can attempt the required intellectual assessment tasks. It is important to note that simply calling a test "nonverbal" does not render the test nonverbal.

Based on the previous operational definition, very few intelligence tests are truly nonverbal. The Test of Nonverbal Intelligence (TONI-III; Brown, Sherbenou, & Johnsen, 1990, 1997), the Comprehensive Test of Nonverbal Intelligence (CTONI; Hammill, Pearson, & Wiederholt, 1996), and the Universal Nonverbal Intelligence Test (UNIT; Bracken & McCallum, 1998) are each administered in a 100% nonverbal fashion. The Leiter International Performance Test–Revised (Leiter-R; Roid & Miller, 1997) is administered in a nonverbal manner with the exception of a few subtests. That is, the revised Leiter requires or advocates the use of verbal directions only rarely among its 20 subtests.

An operational definition is also needed for the term "nonverbal intellectual assessment." Bracken and McCallum (1998) use this term to describe the *process* of assessing the construct of intelligence in a nonverbal fashion. Although other test authors use this term to describe the assessment of a construct called "nonverbal intelligence," "nonverbal reasoning," or "nonverbal abilities" (Brown, Sherbenou, & Johnsen, 1990, 1997; Hammill, Pearson, & Wiederholt, 1996; Naglieri, 1985), Bracken and McCallum (1998) suggest that the central construct assessed by most "nonverbal intelligence tests" is in fact general intelligence. This distinction in terminology is more than a matter of semantics and has implications for how instruments are used with the many diverse populations for which they were intended.

If those intelligence tests that purportedly assess nonverbal intelligence (e.g., TONI-III, CTONI) do in fact assess a construct that is theoretically different from the construct assessed on traditional intelligence tests (i.e., general intelligence), then these tests would be inappropriate for drawing inferences about children's overall intellectual functioning. Such tests should not be used interchangeably with traditional intelligence tests in situations in which decisions about eligibility are made. However, given the strong correlations and comparable mean scores between some nonverbal intelligence tests (e.g., Leiter-R, UNIT) and traditional language-loaded intelligence tests, one could conclude that these instruments do in fact assess the same construct as language-loaded intelligence tests, and that this construct is general intelligence. Several of the most significant nonverbal tests are presented in the Don't Forget (see p. 10).

DISTINCTION BETWEEN UNIDIMENSIONAL AND MULTIDIMENSIONAL TESTS

Among the various nonverbal tests, there are two basic types. Some nonverbal tests assess a narrow aspect of intelligence through the use of progressive ma-

DON'T FORGET

....

Significant Nonverbal Tasks/Tests of Intelligence

Name of Test	Approximate Date of Introduction/Use
1. Seguin Form Board	1907
2. Knox Cube Test	1914
3. Porteus Mazes	1915
4. Kohs Block Design	1919
5. Healy Picture Completion Test	1914, 1918, 1921
6. Army Beta; Beta III	1918, 1921, 1934, 1946, 1999
7. Arthur Point Scale*	1919, 1925
8. Draw A Person	1926
9. Leiter International Performance Scale*	1929, 1948, 1997
10. Raven's Progressive Matrices	1938, 1947, 1956, 1998
11. Culture Fair Intelligence Test	1960
12. Columbia Mental Maturity Scale	1972
13. Test of Nonverbal Intelligence	1980, 1990, 1997
14. Comprehensive Test of Nonverbal Intelligence	1996
15. General Ability Measure for Adults	1997
16. Naglieri Nonverbal Ability Test	1996
17. Universal Nonverbal Intelligence Test*	1998

*Multidimensional tests

trices. Other, more comprehensive nonverbal tests assess multiple facets of examinees' intelligence (e.g., memory, reasoning, attention). While there are numerous progressive matrix tests available, there are only two comprehensive nonverbal tests of intelligence: the UNIT and the Leiter-R. Tests of the matrix solution type include the CTONI, TONI-III, Matrix Analogies Test (MAT; Naglieri, 1985a, 1985b), Naglieri Nonverbal Ability Test (NNAT; Naglieri, 1996), General Ability Measure for Adults (GAMA; Naglieri & Bardos, 1997), and Raven's Progressive Matrices (Raven, Raven, & Court, 1998). Given the narrow focus of the matrix analogy type tests and the fact that many of these tests employ verbal directions, these instruments are best suited for "low stakes" screening applications or in some cases, large scale group assessments (i.e., NNAT). When psychoeducational assessments are conducted for "high stakes" placement, eligibility, or diagnostic decision-making reasons, broader, more comprehensive measures of intelligence would be appropriate (i.e., Leiter-R, UNIT). These more comprehensive tests are are often referred to as "multidimensional" because they include multiple measures of the overall construct of intelligence. That is, they typically include multiple tasks or sub-tests, each designed to assess a different slice of the intelligence pie.

Perhaps the first multidimensional nonverbal test was the Arthur Point Scale of Performance Test, because of its emphasis on including multiple tasks. Currently, only the Leiter-R and the UNIT provide multidimensional nonverbal assessment. Importantly, because multidimensional tests incorporate several measures, they typically have impressive psychometric properties relative to unidimensional tests (e.g., higher correlations with achievement and other broad-based measures of intelligence [Bracken & McCallum, 1998]). In Chapter Two we present a description of the most commonly used individually and group-administered unidimensional ("low stakes") tests, including their developmental and psychometric properties; guidelines for administration, scoring, and clinical interpretation; and strengths and weaknesses. In Chapters Three through Six we review the two comprehensive ("high stakes") nonverbal measures of intelligence. Guidelines for administration, scoring, and clinical interpretation are presented, as are strengths and weaknesses.

SUMMARY

Chapter One presents an overview and outlines the structure of *Essentials of Nonverbal Assessment*. Our goal

=*Rapid Reference 1.3*

Some Salient Distinctions between Unidimensional and Multidimensional Tests

Unidimensional tests assess primarily one facet of intelligence; multidimensional tests assess several facets

Unidimensional tests are used for screening purposes; multidimensional tests are used for placement purposes

Unidimensional tests often predict academic achievement with less power than do multidimensional tests

Unidimensional tests provide less diagnostic information than do multidimensional tests has been to present the rationale for and history of nonverbal assessment, with a particular focus on the developments since the early 1900s. One of the strongest early motivations for the development of nonverbal measures emerged as a result of the practical needs associated with personnel selection in wartime. Because many potential soldiers had received little formal education and because the country was becoming increasingly diverse during this period, many recruits were illiterate, foreign-born, or both. These individuals could not be assessed with traditional language-loaded tests. Similar needs were being expressed in the private sector during the first half of the twentieth century. In addition, psychologists and other health care specialists began to demand more sophisticated measures for use with language-impaired individuals with central nervous system trauma, psychiatric diagnoses, and so on. Nonverbal tests were developed to meet these needs.

Most recently, two major types of nonverbal tests have been developed: unidimensional or "low stakes" tests, and more comprehensive "high stakes" multidimensional tests. Chapters Two through Six describe the theory, psychometric properties, administration/scoring/interpretation guidelines, and strengths and weaknesses of the most commonly used group- and individually-administered nonverbal tests, including those described as unidimensional and multidimensional.

🐿 TEST YOURSELF 🐿

1. **The Army Alpha test was used to**
   (a) Assess recruits who could read
   (b) Assess recruits who could not read
   (c) Assess recruits who wanted to specialize in nonverbal code breaking
   (d) Assess only female recruits who could not read

2. **Wechsler included which one of the following existing tests into the WISC-III?**
   (a) Kohs Block Design
   (b) Cattell's Picture Vocabulary
   (c) Seguin's Form Board Test
   (d) Kaufman's Matrix Analogies Test

3. **The Army Beta test was used to**
   - (a) Assess only females who could read
   - (b) Assess recruits who wanted to specialize in language-based code breaking
   - (c) Assess recruits who could not read
   - (d) Assess all recruits who could read

4. **Which one of the following is a multidimensional test?**
   - (a) Comprehensive Test of Nonverbal Intelligence
   - (b) Matrix Analogies Test
   - (c) Test of Nonverbal Intelligence–Third Edition
   - (d) Universal Nonverbal Intelligence Test

5. **Unidimensional tests are best for making _____ decisions**
   - (a) Placement
   - (b) Diagnostic
   - (c) Screening
   - (d) Intervention

6. **Which of the following might be considered the first multidimensional nonverbal test?**
   - (a) UNIT
   - (b) Arthur Point Scale of Performance Tests
   - (c) Leiter
   - (d) Healy Picture Completion Test

7. **One of the first documented cases to make use of nonverbal assessment was the "Wild Boy of Aveyron," and was conducted by**
   - (a) Jean Piaget
   - (b) Jean Itard
   - (c) Henri Binet
   - (d) Paul Simon

8. **As a psychologist charged with making a placement decision for culturally different children, you should choose which of the following nonverbal tests?**
   - (a) UNIT
   - (b) CTONI
   - (c) TONI-III
   - (d) WISC-PIQ

(continued)

9. According to Frijda and Jahoda (1966) it has not been possible to develop a totally culture-free test because

   (a) Language is a window to the intellect; all tests need to include a language component

   (b) Nonverbal, culture-free tests cannot predict achievement very well

   (c) There are too many diverse cultures

   (d) All tests are anchored in an originating culture

10. With over 200 languages spoken, the city of _____ may be the most culturally diverse in the United States.

   (a) Atlanta

   (b) Boston

   (c) Los Angeles

   (d) Chicago

Answers: 1. a; 2. a; 3. c; 4. d; 5. c; 6. b; 7. b; 8. a; 9. d; 10. d

Two

UNIDIMENSIONAL NONVERBAL TESTS

In the previous chapter, the uses and applications of unidimensional and multidimensional tests were described. Multidimensional tests offer advantages of increased assessment breadth and comprehensiveness, but require individual administration. In contrast, tests that are unidimensional in theoretical orientation have narrower breadth but are often suitable for screening applications and group administration, thereby permitting more efficient administration and scoring. In this chapter, six relatively unidimensional nonverbal tests are described. All of these measures may be individually administered, but four of the tests were normed in a group format and accordingly are suitable for group administration. The constructs that each test purports to measure are listed in Rapid Reference 2.1.

Each of these measures may be used in varying degrees to assess general cognitive and intellectual ability, to screen students potentially eligible for special services, to more fairly assess students with limited English proficiency or with diverse cultural and educational backgrounds, to screen students who would be disadvantaged by traditional language-loaded assessments (e.g., deaf students), and to assess what students *can* do despite whatever language, motor, or color-vision limitations they may have. These instruments may also be useful in identifying intellectually gifted students.

Four of the measures discussed in this chapter are suitable for use with school-aged children: the Comprehensive Test of Nonverbal Intelligence (CTONI; Hammill, Pearson, & Wiederholt, 1996), the Naglieri Nonverbal Ability Test (NNAT; Naglieri, 1996), the Raven's Progressive Matrices (RPM; Raven, Raven, & Court, 1998), and the Test of Nonverbal Intelligence (TONI-III; Brown, Sherbenou, & Johnsen, 1997). Five of the measures may be used with adults: the Beta III (Kellogg & Morton, 1999), the CTONI (Hammill, Pearson, & Wiederholt, 1996), the General Ability Measure for

≡ *Rapid Reference 2.1*

What the Unidimensional Nonverbal Tests Purport to Measure

Beta III	nonverbal intellectual ability, "including visual information processing, processing speed, spatial and nonverbal reasoning, and aspects of fluid intelligence" (Kellogg & Morton, 1999, p. 1)
CTONI	"those particular abilities that exist independently of language and that increase a person's capacity to function intelligently" (Hammill, Pearson, & Wiederholt, 1996, p. 1)
GAMA	general ability, i.e., "the application of reasoning and logic to solve problems" (Naglieri & Bardos, 1997, p. 1)
NNAT	general ability
RPM	eductive ability, i.e., the ability to forge new insights, the ability to discern meaning in confusion, the ability to perceive, and the ability to identify relationships (Raven, Raven, & Court, 1998)
TONI-III	"abstract/figural problem solving" (Brown, Sherbenou, & Johnsen, 1997, p. 28)

Adults (GAMA; Naglieri & Bardos, 1997), the Raven's Progressive Matrices (Raven, Raven, & Court, 1998), and the TONI-III (Brown, Sherbenou, & Johnsen, 1997).

In general, group-administered unidimensional tests have several advantages over individually-administered tests—cost effectiveness, ease of administration, and testing efficiency—while usually providing a good estimate of overall nonverbal intellectual ability. However, these benefits should be measured against several limitations: (a) dependence on brief language-based administrative instructional sets (i.e., most unidimensional nonverbal tests have verbal directions), sometimes requiring one or more different translated instructions; (b) predominantly unidimensional testing formats, which restrict the types of cognitive abilities assessed; (c) the absence of adaptive testing

DON'T FORGET

Unidimensional nonverbal tests offer the benefit of assessment efficiency in comparison to a more time-consuming comprehensive assessment. Think about your reasons for testing.

formats that permit differential starting points and discontinuation rules that are sensitive to examinees' different ability levels; (d) limited potential to adapt test administration procedures to the needs of individuals with handicapping conditions or disabilities; (e) limited profiling capabilities of cognitive strengths and weaknesses; (f) limited use with preschool and early school-aged children who are less adept at group testing; and (g) the inability to assess important cognitive dimensions such as memory, which are less conducive to group testing than to individually-administered tests. In general, group-administered nonverbal tests serve as good screeners for children who are at risk or of low ability, but these instruments have seriously limited flexibility and limited validity in predicting real-life outcomes.

In the following section, each of the unidimensional nonverbal measures is described, along with its developmental history, including prior editions. Essential elements of administration, scoring, and interpretation are presented, followed by a description of the instrument's strengths and weaknesses relative to test standardization, psychometric properties including reliability and validity, test fairness, and the ease of test administration.

BETA III

The Beta III (Kellogg & Morton, 1999) is a group-administered test for adults between the ages of 16 and 89 years. It is intended to measure visual information processing, processing speed, spatial and nonverbal reasoning, and aspects of fluid intelligence. Beta III consists of five tests and requires approximately 25–30 minutes to administer. The test is intended for use with individuals who are non-English speakers, illiterate, or language-disordered, or for other individuals for whom nonverbal assessment would be most appropriate, such as individuals in correctional facilities or unskilled laborers.

The Beta III originated in the Group Beta Examination (Yerkes, 1921) developed by the U.S. Army to assess the intelligence of illiterate and non-English speaking recruits during World War I (Thorndike & Lohman, 1990). The Army Beta was a nonverbal counterpart to the verbally loaded Army Alpha and included the tasks that Wechsler later adapted to become the Coding and Digit Symbol subtests of the Wechsler intelligence scales. A subsequent adaptation of the Beta (Kellogg & Morton, 1934) made the test suitable for civilian applications, and it was later restandardized and reformatted by Lindner and Gurvitz (1946) to more closely resemble the leading intelligence scales of its day. A major revision and update of item content, as well as collection of a new normative sample, were undertaken in 1978 for the second edition. The revision that resulted in the Beta III improved its content, updated norms, extended the instrument's age range, and raised the ceiling to an IQ of 155 points.

Administration

The administration directions for all five tests are verbal, require about 10 to 15 minutes in total duration, and are available in English and Spanish. The time required to complete the test once the directions are complete is about 14.5 minutes. In total, the Beta III requires approximately 25 to 30 minutes to administer.

The Beta III is typically administered in small groups and requires at least one proctor for every 15 examinees. Directions for administration may be read directly from the *Beta III Manual*. The proctor is instructed to read the directions slowly and clearly, and the proctor must have a stopwatch or similar timing device to ensure compliance with time limits. The spoken directions are sufficiently complex that they should be reviewed in advance. In several instances, the proctor must display sample pages that are folded back or special figures (e.g., the not equal sign, ≠), so the setting should enable the proctor to move freely among examinees with materials that can be easily seen. Directions, practice problems, and feedback are provided for every test. There are opportunities for proctors to answer examinees' questions and to provide feedback.

There are five Beta III tests, several of which will be familiar to users of other major intelligence tests:

Coding. The examinee writes numbers that correspond to a symbol, based upon a number-symbol key provided at the top of the page.
Picture Completion. The examinee draws a missing part to complete a picture.
Clerical Checking. The examinee circles an equal sign (=) or not equal sign (≠) to indicate whether pairs of pictures, geometric figures, or number strings are the same or different.

Picture Absurdities. The examinee places an X on the one picture out of four that illustrates an object or event that is wrong or foolish.

Matrix Reasoning. The examinee selects the one of five choices that best completes a 2 × 2 matrix with three figures and a missing element.

Individuals with special needs or those for whom the instructions are too complex may require separate individualized administration. The time limits and scoring characteristics of each test appear in Rapid Reference 2.2.

Scoring and Interpretation

Items completed by the examinee within the time limits on the Beta III are scored with a scoring key and require minimal subjective evaluation by the examiner. Three of the tests are either multiple or dichotomous choice formats; Coding requires writing the number corresponding to the symbol, and Picture

≡ *Rapid Reference 2.2*

Beta III Test Characteristics

Beta III Tests	Time Limit	Format	Raw Score Range	Scoring
Coding	120 seconds	Correct number written	0 to 140	1 point per correct response
Picture Completion	150 seconds	Correct element drawn	0 to 24	1 point per correct response
Clerical Checking	120 seconds	Dichotomous choice	≤ −11 to 55	Number of correct items minus number of errors
Picture Absurdities	180 seconds	Multiple choice	0 to 24	1 point per correct response
Matrix Reasoning	300 seconds	Multiple choice	0 to 25	1 point per correct response

Completion requires drawing. Artistic accuracy is not evaluated for Picture Completion.

The Beta III yields age-correct scaled scores (Mean = 10, Standard Deviation = 3) and an overall Beta III IQ (M = 100, SD = 15), as well as percentile ranks and confidence intervals at 90% and 95% confidence. The Beta III IQ and percentile ranks do not, however, reflect the same absolute level of performance from individuals in different age groups, since they are based on the theoretical values for a normal distribution and may vary according to the degree to which the performance of the sample deviated from normal curve expectations.

The test is best interpreted at the composite level, although factor analyses suggest that three tests (Matrix Reasoning, Picture Completion, and Picture Absurdities) assess nonverbal reasoning, while two tests (Coding and Clerical Checking) measure processing speed. Accordingly, divergent findings for these groups of tests may be appropriate for interpretation, although the manual does not explicitly describe a methodology for making comparisons between the two factors. The authors recommend *against* interpretation of individual Beta III tests.

Strengths and Weaknesses

This section presents several strengths and weaknesses of the Beta III. In general, the principal strengths of the Beta III include its ease of use, high correlations with other indices of intelligence, and exemplary standardization sample. Limitations include inconsistent presentations of construct validity (i.e., one dimension of cognitive ability or two?), the absence of test reliability studies, and minimal coverage of test bias. Rapid Reference 2.3 summarizes the Beta III's strengths and weaknesses.

Ease of Use

Given the brevity of its administration, its group-administration format, and use of scoring keys, the Beta III is a relatively easy test to use. Because the Beta III must be hand scored, the test requires slightly more interpretive effort than other multiple choice machine scored tests for adults, such as the GAMA. However, the required examination of the individual's actual responses also increases the likelihood that clinically meaningful information

≡ *Rapid Reference 2.3*

Beta III Strengths and Weaknesses

Strengths	Weaknesses
• Brief and easy to use	• Construct validity (one factor or two?)
• Inclusion of practice problems	
• English and Spanish directions	• Pervasive timing or speed requirements
• Well-normed, highly representative standardization sample	• Low ceilings for selected tests
• Good convergent validity with other intelligence tests	• Constituent tests have inadequate reliabilities
	• Insufficient coverage of test fairness and bias

may be derived from examinee errors or other examinee response characteristics.

The inclusion of both English and Spanish administration directions enhances the use of the Beta III across the two most dominant languages in the United States, but the verbal instructions are somewhat lengthy and contain many potentially difficult words (e.g., "prong," "overlapping," "hacksaw"). The examiner's manual does not report whether these more difficult words have been screened for level of oral comprehension. All Beta III tests are timed or have speed requirements, making the Beta III inappropriate for use with motorically handicapped examinees. The instrument's psychomotor demands are moderately high for the Coding and Picture Completion tests, but minimal for the Clerical Checking, Picture Absurdities, and Matrix Reasoning tests.

A significant asset of the Beta III is its inclusion of multiple practice problems and explanations describing how to complete problems. While adding to the verbiage of this ostensibly nonverbal test, the explanations help to ensure that all examinees know what is expected for each test.

DON'T FORGET

The Beta III IQ may be significantly depressed for motorically impaired examinees because of the heavy dependence on speeded and psychomotorically demanding tests.

Selected Technical Features

The Beta III standardization sample was collected in 1997 and 1998 from a nationally representative sample of 1,260 individuals between the ages of 16 and 89 years, inclusive. The sample was stratified by age, sex, race/ethnicity, educational level, and geographic region. Participants were screened for psychiatric and neurological conditions, including drug or alcohol dependency. An examination of the representativeness of the sample suggests that the Beta III standardization sample closely matches the 1997 U.S. population, with the sample composition rarely deviating by more than two or three percentage points from the U.S. population parameters.

The only form of reliability available for the Beta III is test-retest reliability. Also, stability of the Beta III is presented only for the overall IQ, with test-retest intervals ranging from 2 to 12 weeks. The average stability coefficient, corrected for restriction of range, for the Beta III IQ is .91, with little variability across three age bands. This overall composite stability is fully adequate, but the failure of the test manual to report stability coefficients for individual subtests suggests that the subtests have only limited interpretive value in isolation: "Reliability coefficients are not provided for separate subtests because only the *overall* IQ or percentile has demonstrated sufficient reliability and validity for meaningful interpretation" (Kellog & Morton, 1999, p. 25). Accordingly, the technical properties support the conceptualization of the Beta III as a unidimensional measure despite its multiple subtests, each of which yields scaled score equivalents.

The Beta III IQs range from 48 to 155, and most subtests similarly appear to have adequate floors and ceilings. The exceptions are Picture Absurdities, which has a maximum scaled score equivalent of 14 (+1.33 SD) for most young adults, and Matrix Reasoning, which has a highest possible scaled score equivalent of 15 or 16 (+1.67 to +2.00 SD) for adults ages 16 through 24 years. The implication of this limitation is that IQs among young adults may be disproportionately low due to the requirements of the speeded subtests, such as Coding and Clerical Checking. Floors appear thoroughly adequate on the Beta III, consistent with the test's historical emphasis on testing low ability adults.

Fairness

The test manual provides only a cursory examination of test fairness. Test items from the Beta III that were considered to be potentially biased from a cultural or social point of view were deleted and replaced with new items. The test manual contains a list of external reviewers who likely addressed issues of bias and sensitivity, although the test manual does not explicitly describe this process. No psychometric analyses of test bias, such as differential item functioning (DIF) studies, are reported in the test manual. Insofar as the Beta III is intended for use in correctional facilities, which are inhabited by a disproportionately high number of individuals from racial and ethnic minorities, the absence of a detailed analysis of test fairness is conspicuous.

Validity

Kellogg and Morton (1999) report about a dozen validity studies for the Beta III. In general, these studies suggest that the Beta III correlates highly with other measures of general ability, while tapping more than one underlying dimension of cognitive ability. However, the test manual recommends against interpretation of more than one factor.

Convergent validity studies are reported between the Beta III and the WAIS-III, Raven Standard Progressive Matrices, and several other instruments. In the WAIS-III study, the Beta III and the WAIS-III were administered in counterbalanced order to 182 adults, with an average testing interval of about three to four weeks. When the correlations are corrected for restriction of range and are averaged across samples, the correlations between the Beta III IQ and WAIS-III were .67 for the Verbal IQ, .80 for the Performance IQ, and .77 for the Full Scale IQ. These findings are commensurate with expectations that the Beta III is more strongly related to Performance IQ than Verbal IQ. The authors note that Beta IQ is generally three to four points lower than the WAIS-III FSIQ and PIQ, suggesting that the score differences might be due to sampling error or differences in the abilities assessed by the two instruments. Correlations between the Beta III and the Raven Standard Progressive Matrices (SPM) are based on a counterbalanced administration to a sample of 32 adults. When corrected for restriction of range, the Beta III IQ correlates with the SPM at .75. Weaker correlations are reported for results from screening batteries and other instruments with primary industrial applications (e.g., those reflecting mechanical aptitudes).

Both exploratory and confirmatory factor analyses were conducted on the Beta III and are reported in the examiner's manual. Exploratory factor analyses using principal components analysis with oblique rotation at the subtest level suggest that two major factors account for test performance. The first factor is labeled Nonverbal Reasoning and has primary loadings by the Matrix Reasoning, Picture Completion, and Picture Absurdities subtests. The second factor is labeled Processing Speed and has primary loadings by the Coding and Clerical Checking subtests. Confirmatory factor analyses testing the relative fit of three different models suggest that a two-factor model fits the data better than either a one-factor or a three-factor model. The authors interpret these findings as suggesting that the "Beta III contains two factors" (p. 33), although the test is not structured in a manner to facilitate interpretation of these two factors, and elsewhere the test manual concludes "only the overall IQ or percentile has demonstrated sufficient reliability and validity for meaningful interpretation" (p. 25).

Several special population studies are reported in the *Beta III Manual*, including samples of incarcerated adults (*n* = 388), adults diagnosed with mental retardation (*n* = 68), and adults diagnosed with Attention Deficit Hyperactivity Disorder (ADHD) (*n* = 22). In the sample of individuals in correctional settings, the mean Beta III performance fell fully within the average range for each of five age groups, a finding somewhat at odds with expectations that inmates tend to perform below average on measures of intelligence. The authors qualify results by noting that the prison sample was a convenience sample that is not necessarily representative of the general prison population. In the investigation of individuals with mental retardation, results showed that 79% of individuals diagnosed with mild mental retardation obtained Beta III IQ scores from 56 to 70 points, and 63% of individuals diagnosed with moderate mental retardation obtained Beta III IQ scores of 55 points or less. The authors conclude that the Beta III is sensitive but not specific to a diagnosis of mental retardation, that is, that it correctly diagnoses individuals with mental retardation but may incorrectly suggest a diagnosis of mental retardation in individuals who should not be so classified. The investigation of adults diagnosed with ADHD compared with a demographically matched comparison group from the standardization sample yielded modest overall IQ differences, with the largest subtest

≋Rapid Reference 2.4

Beta III

Authors: C. E. Kellogg and N. W. Morton
Publication date: 1999
What the test measures: Visual information processing, processing speed, spatial and nonverbal reasoning, and aspects of fluid intelligence
Age range: 16 to 89
Administration format: Group or individual
Administration time: 25–30 minutes
Qualifications of examiners: Individuals with a bachelor's degree in psychology, education, counseling, speech therapy, or occupational therapy may administer the Beta III
Publisher: The Psychological Corporation

discrepancies concentrated primarily on the subtests tapping processing speed.

See Rapid Reference 2.4 for general information about the Beta III.

COMPREHENSIVE TEST OF NONVERBAL INTELLIGENCE

The Comprehensive Test of Nonverbal Intelligence (CTONI; Hammill, Pearson, & Wiederholt, 1996) is an individually-administered, six subtest, matrix-formatted test that purports to provide a comprehensive measure of "nonverbal intelligence" for children, adolescents, and adults between the ages of 6 and 90 years. The CTONI typically requires one hour to administer and yields a Nonverbal Intelligence Quotient (NIQ), a Pictorial Nonverbal Intelligence Quotient (PNIQ), and a Geometric Nonverbal Intelligence Quotient (GNIQ). All subtests utilize a matrix-based, multiple choice format and require pointing by the examinee to indicate correct responses.

In the CTONI, *nonverbal intelligence* is defined as "those particular abilities that exist independently of language and that increase a person's capacity to function intelligently." (Hammill, Pearson, & Wiederholt, 1996, p. 1). This perspective differs from the conventional wisdom that nonverbal tests assess *general intelligence* through nonverbal assessment procedures, rather than a distinctive form of intelligence in itself. The CTONI utilizes a design that includes subtests that assess analogical reasoning, categorical classifications, and sequential reasoning in two different contexts: pictures of familiar objects (e.g., people and animals) and abstract geometric designs.

Administration

Based upon the test design of two types of stimuli (pictures and geometric designs), each applied across three abilities (analogical reasoning, categorical classifications, and sequential reasoning), the CTONI offers six subtests: Pictorial Analogies, Geometric Analogies, Pictorial Categories, Geometric Categories, Pictorial Sequences, and Geometric Sequences. The easel book format makes this test suitable only for individual administration.

Subtests may be administered orally to students who speak English, or in pantomime to those who speak a language other than English or who are deaf or language-impaired. It is unclear whether the test was normed and standardized with both administration procedures or only the oral presentation, as only one set of norms is presented. A single study purports to demonstrate that the oral and pantomime administration formats yield equivalent results. Stability coefficients for 33 third-grade students and 30 11th-grade students who were given the pantomimed instructions and then retested with oral instructions in approximately one month yielded negligible mean score differences for both subtests and composite scales. Across the two grade levels, subtest "stability" (i.e., delayed alternate-form reliability) coefficients ranged from .79 to .89; the composite score stability coefficients ranged from .88 to .94. The use of a test-retest stability study to demonstrate the equivalency of administration formats is unconventional, because it combines and confounds demonstration of construct stability (i.e., test-retest reliability) with two alternate-form administration modes (i.e., alternate-form reliability).

A brief description of each subtest and its administration procedure follows:

> *Pictorial Analogies (PA).* PA employs a two-by-two matrix format that presents a pictorial analogy (e.g., apple is to tree as grape is to . . .

vine) that is to be completed by the examinee. The examiner points to each of the elements in the first row of the matrix to identify the relationship between the two objects pictured. Next, the examiner points to the first picture in the second row, then points to the empty space adjacent to the pictured object. The empty space in the second row is to be completed by one of the five pictures depicted below. In this subtest the examinee is expected "to understand that *this* is to *that* . . . as *this* is to *what* . . . ?" (Hammill, Pearson, & Wiederholt, 1996, p. 8).

Geometric Analogies (GA). GA employs the same two-by-two matrix format as PA, but GA presents geometric figures rather than pictorial stimuli. The GA subtest requires the examinee to discern that *this* object is to *that* object . . . as *this* object is to *which* of the following objects?

Pictorial Categories (PC). The PC subtest uses an item type that presents "an association format to intuit relationships and to construct categories" (Hammill, Pearson, & Wiederholt, 1996, p. 8). Examinees are expected to select which pictured object most closely relates to the stimulus objects presented in the incomplete matrix. For example, an item might present two unique automobiles side-by-side, and the correct response would be another automobile that is selected from among five different non-category inclusive vehicles (e.g., truck, motorcycle, bus).

Geometric Categories (GC). GC employs the same administration format as PC, but in GC geometric designs, rather than pictured objects, are used to create associations and categories (e.g., squares selected from among other common geometric figures).

Pictorial Sequences (PS). PS includes problem-solving tasks that employ pictured objects that are presented within the format of a progressive sequence. For example, three stimulus pictures might depict a large ball, a medium-sized ball, a smaller ball, and a blank square. Below the incomplete sequence would be presented several different sized balls, with only one ball being smaller than the ball that was depicted last in the stimulus sequence (i.e., the *smallest* ball).

Geometric Sequences (GS). GS uses the same administration format as PS, but GS uses abstract geometric designs instead of pictured objects to depict developing sequences (e.g., an arrow that rotates 45 degrees in each of three successive squares).

The sole response modality required of the examinee by the CTONI is selecting the correct response from an array of choices and pointing to it. No oral responses, reading, writing, or object manipulation are required.

A computer-administered pay-per-use adaptation known as the CTONI-CA is also available. The computer provides verbal instructions and visual presentation of test stimuli to the examinee, who then responds by using the mouse to indicate the correct response. The CTONI-CA offers automated discontinuation of subtests after the examinee reaches a ceiling, computation of all scores, and generation of an automated score report that can be imported into word processing software programs.

Scoring

Within the multiple choice format, all items are scored dichotomously as either passed or failed, and are summed within each subtest to generate a subtest scaled score (M = 10; SD = 3). Scores are then summed across the geometric item types and pictorial item types to produce two subscales, a Pictorial Nonverbal Intelligence Quotient (PNIQ) and a Geometric Nonverbal Intelligence Quotient (GNIQ), and a total test composite score labeled the Nonverbal Intelligence Quotient (NIQ), each with a mean of 100 and a standard deviation of 15. In addition to standard scores, the CTONI produces percentile ranks, age equivalents, and descriptive classifications.

Interpretation

The CTONI produces six subtest scores, two subscales, and a total test score for interpretive purposes. Interpreting the CTONI is straightforward and should begin with the total test score, the Nonverbal Intelligence Quotient (NIQ). The NIQ is the most reliable score and best represents the examinee's overall test performance. Examiners may also wish to examine any differences that exist between the examinee's Pictorial Nonverbal Intelligence Quotient (PNIQ) and Geometric Nonverbal Intelligence Quotient (GNIQ) to draw inferences about the examinee's ability to solve concrete versus abstract reasoning problems.

≡Rapid Reference 2.5

CTONI Strengths and Weaknesses

Strengths	Weaknesses
• Simplicity and ease of administration	• Construct validity (insufficient support for pictorial and geometric composite indices)
• Availability of computerized administration	• Questionable interpretive yield for hour-long test administration duration
• Nationally representative normative sample	
• Good subtest reliabilities	
• Promising preliminary evidence of test fairness	

Strengths and Weaknesses

This section presents several strengths and weaknesses of the CTONI (summarized in Rapid Reference 2.5). In general, the principal strengths of the CTONI include its ease of use and several technical characteristics, such as its normative sample and test reliabilities. Demonstration of mean test performances across gender and racial/ethnic groups also suggests that fairness may represent an area of possible strength for the CTONI, although the studies suggesting this conclusion suffer from methodological limitations. These strengths must be balanced against problems with the test's validity and interpretive yield, given its lengthy (for a unidimensional nonverbal cognitive test) hour-long administration time.

Ease of Use

The CTONI is very easy to administer, due to its brief verbal instructions, matrix-based administration format, and multiple choice pointing response format. Its simplicity explains why the test is amenable to automated computer administration and a simple point-and-click response by the examinee.

Selected Technical Features

Several technical features of the CTONI represent areas of strength. These include the normative sample and the high score reliabilities. At the same time, the CTONI shows some evidence of an insufficient ceiling for adolescents beyond age 13.

The CTONI was standardized and normed on a sample of 2,129 children and adolescents residing in 23 states. The normative sample was selected according to the following demographic characteristics: geographic region, gender, race, residence (i.e., urban, rural), ethnicity, family income, educational attainment of parents, and disability status. When the normative sample and the U.S. population are compared to assess sampling accuracy for the total sample, all selection variables reflect the U.S. population parameters fairly well (i.e., generally within 3 to 4 percentage points).

Indices of scale and subtest internal score consistency (coefficient *alpha*) tend to be high on the CTONI. Across 13 normative age groups, the NIQ produced an average reliability coefficient of .97; the PNIQ produced an average reliability coefficient of .93; and the GNIQ average alpha was .95. Average reliabilities for the six CTONI subtests range from .86 to .92. Accordingly, the CTONI shows evidence of high levels of internal consistency at both the subtest and composite score levels. Coefficient alphas for various subsets of the standardization sample, including samples of individuals described as "Caucasoid," African American, American Indian, Asian, Panamanian, ESL, learning disabled, deaf, male, and female, are reported and tend to be comparable to those obtained for the entire standardization sample, suggesting that test score reliabilities are comparable and reliable for these various groups.

The CTONI examiner's manual also provides correlational data between subtest raw scores and examinees' chronological age. Correlations range from .45 and .66 for the 13 age groups, and importantly, the tabled data also reveal that the CTONI evidences virtually no growth after age 13. Between the ages of 13 and 18 years, only one to three items distinguish the various age levels, which suggests that the CTONI lacks considerable ceiling after age 13.

Fairness

Studies of test bias and fairness reported in the CTONI examiner's manual include Differential Item Functioning (DIF) analyses and group mean score comparisons. DIF studies were conducted according to gender, combined race/ethnicity/language (i.e., African Americans, ESL students, American Indians), and disability (i.e., learning disabled students). At least one item was found to be psychometrically biased within the test for each group; however, there were from one to five biased items identified for each sample studied. Comparison of group mean score differences for examinees with various demographic characteristics yielded only minor variation from the standardization normative mean of 100. For example, both Hispanics and African Americans earned group mean NIQs of 97. However, children and adolescents who were identified as deaf earned a mean NIQ that was 10 points lower than the normative mean, and ESL students earned a mean NIQ that was 8 points lower than the normative mean. However, these studies of group mean score differences are constrained by a serious methodological limitation. No evidence is presented that the groups are comparable on any meaningful demographic or stratification variables (e.g., socioeconomic status); therefore, comparisons of group mean scores may yield misleading conclusions. Interpretation of these fairness studies should be considered very cautiously, and additional studies employing matched samples must be conducted to control for these potentially confounding extraneous variables.

Validity

Given that the CTONI takes approximately one hour to administer, there must be demonstrated value in the design of the test and the constructs it purports to measure. The validity of the distinction between the PNIQ and GNIQ is, however, unsupported at this time. An exploratory factor analysis conducted on the CTONI standardization sample yielded a one-factor solution, and similarly, a one-factor solution was reported for several demographically different subgroups (e.g., males, females, Hispanics, American Indians).

Criterion-related concurrent validity studies reported in the examiner's manual also show that higher correlations exist between the CTONI, a nonverbal intelligence test, and the WISC-III Verbal Scale than between the CTONI and the WISC-III Performance Scale. The first study correlated the CTONI, the WISC-III, and the TONI-II for a sample of 43 students in Dallas, Texas, who were previously identified as learning disabled. After correcting the validity coefficients for attenuation due to imperfect test reliability, the authors

DON'T FORGET

The value of interpreting discrepancies between Pictorial and Geometric nonverbal intelligence on the CTONI is as yet undemonstrated. Use appropriate caution.

=== Rapid Reference 2.6

Comprehensive Test of Nonverbal Intelligence (CTONI)

Authors: D. D. Hammill, N. A. Pearson, and J. L. Wiederholt
Publication date: 1996
What the test measures: Nonverbal intelligence and reasoning ability
Age range: 6 to 90
Administration format: Individual
Administration time: 60 minutes
Qualifications of examiners: Individuals with some formal training in mental ability assessment, including test statistics, administration, scoring, and interpretation; supervised practice is desirable
Publisher: Pro-Ed

reported concurrent validity coefficients of .64, .66, and .81 between the WISC-III Full Scale IQ and the PNIQ, GNIQ, and NIQ, respectively. Concurrent validity coefficients of this magnitude provide only moderate support for the contention that the test measures intelligence. Ironically, the three CTONI composites correlated more highly with the WISC-III Verbal IQ (i.e., .59, .56, .76) than with the Performance IQ (i.e., .51, .55, .70).

The second criterion-related study involved the administration of the WISC-III Performance Scale and the CTONI to 32 deaf students from two other cities in Texas. In this instance the correlations were corrected for both restriction in range *and* attenuation for imperfect reliability. In this study, the twice-corrected correlations between the CTONI PNIQ, GNIQ, and NIQ and the WISC-III PIQ were .87, .85, and .90, respectively. In neither study did the authors provide the means or standard deviations for the predictor or criterion measures or the uncorrected coefficients, so it is impossible to determine the extent to which these tests produce comparable scores in actual use.

Summary information about the CTONI appears in Rapid Reference 2.6.

GENERAL ABILITY MEASURE FOR ADULTS (GAMA)

The General Ability Measure for Adults (GAMA; Naglieri & Bardos, 1997) is a self-administered, four subtest, multiple choice test that assesses overall general ability for adults 18 years of age and older. The GAMA requires 25 minutes to administer and yields a GAMA IQ and subtest scaled scores for four subtests: Matching, Sequences, Analogies, and Construction.

The 66 items of the GAMA have been designed to "require the application of reasoning and logic to solve problems that exclusively use abstract designs and shapes" (Naglieri & Bardos, 1997, p. 1). Items appear in the same blue, yellow, white, and black format as the older Matrix Analogies Test (MAT; Naglieri, 1985a, 1985b).

Administration

There are four sets of directions for the administration of the GAMA, depending on whether the test is self- or group-administered and whether the examiner uses a self-scoring or scannable answer document. In most administrations, GAMA instructions are read by examinees. The instructions are written at a 2.4 grade level and are available in English and Spanish.

The test begins with four sample items that present each of the four item types. After completing the sample items, examinees are given 25 minutes to complete the items presented in the stimulus book. For each item, the examinee is required to indicate which of six choices completes a pattern. The GAMA consists of four subtests, each having distinctive item types.

Matching. Items in this subtest require examination of the shapes and colors of a stimulus to determine which of the response options is identical.

Sequences. Items require the analysis of the interrelationships of designs as they move successively through space; the examinee must select the response option that completes the sequence.

Analogies. Items involve the discovery of the relationships in a pair of abstract figures and the recognition of similar conceptual relationships in a different pair of figures.

Construction. Items require the analysis, synthesis, and rotation of spatial designs to construct a new figure.

These subtests parallel the four types of items appearing in the MAT (Naglieri, 1985a, 1985b) and the NNAT (Naglieri, 1997).

Scoring and Interpretation

The GAMA multiple choice items are scored as correct or incorrect. Materials may be hand-scored or machine-scored.

GAMA yields a total test standard score, labeled the GAMA IQ, based on the four subtest scaled scores, with a mean of 100 and a standard deviation of 15. A 90% confidence interval may also be generated, as well as percentile ranks and a descriptive classification ranging from Well Below Average to Very Superior.

The four subtest scaled scores each has a mean of 10 and a standard deviation of 3. Subtest scores include descriptive classifications and strength/weakness profiling.

Strengths and Weaknesses

In this section, as well as Rapid Reference 2.7, strengths and weaknesses of the GAMA are described. The major strengths of the GAMA include its ease of use and flexible administration options. Its normative sample is nationally representative, and its convergent validity with other intelligence tests is good. Limitations include marginal reliabilities at the subtest level and insufficient coverage of test fairness and psychometric bias after items were originally screened during test development for bias. In addition, the GAMA's literacy requirements may lead many examiners to consider other administration options for poorly educated samples.

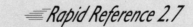

Rapid Reference 2.7

GAMA Strengths and Weaknesses

Strengths	Weaknesses
• Brief and easy to use	• Literacy requirements for most common administration option
• Self- or group-administration options	• Marginal subtest reliabilities
• Computer scoring is available	• Insufficient coverage of test fairness and bias
• Rigorous and representative normative sample	
• Good convergent validity with other intelligence tests	

Ease of Use

The self- or group-administration format, available in English or Spanish, makes the GAMA easy to use. Its 25-minute duration keeps administration brief and its computer scoring options expedite scoring. Its reading requirements, however, distinguish it as the only individually-administered test requiring literacy on the part of the examinee. Administration options are available for examinees who cannot read.

Selected Technical Features

This section summarizes selected technical aspects of the GAMA, including a relatively rigorous normative standardization sample and high correlations with other measures of intelligence. Reliability coefficients are generally adequate at the overall IQ level but not at the subtest level.

GAMA was normed on a national sample of 2,360 adults partitioned into 11 age groups. Stratifying variables for the normative sample included age, gender, race/ethnic group, educational level, and geographic region. The oldest age level, 75 years and older, was the only sampled age group that experienced significant deviation from the national population in terms of region of the U.S., with some discrepancies of approximately 8%. Gender, race/ethnicity, and educational level variables also had a fairly good match with the U.S. population at independent age levels, with only minor (2% to 5%) discrepancies between the GAMA sample and the U.S. population on these variables.

Split-half reliability coefficients are reported for the four item types and the GAMA IQ for the entire standardization sample. Reliabilities for the GAMA IQ across the 11 age levels ranged from .79 to .94, with seven of the age levels reporting reliabilities at or above .90. The average total test split-half reliability was .90 across all age levels. Average reliabilities for the four item types are marginal at .65, .66, .79, and .81 for the Construction, Matching, Sequences, and Analogies items, respectively.

Test-retest reliability was investigated using a sample of 86 adults that, while not representative of the population, was broadly represented according to gender, race/ethnicity, and educational level. With a mean test-retest interval of 25 days and a range of two to six weeks, the GAMA IQ produced a stability coefficient of .67. The four item types produced test-retest correlations that ranged from .38 (Construction) to .74 (Sequences). Gain scores of slightly less than one-third of a standard deviation were consistent across the item types and GAMA IQ.

Fairness

All items were examined during early stages of test development with the Mantel-Haenzel statistical procedure for detecting differential item function (DIF) between males and females, and whites and nonwhites. Items yielding evidence of DIF were removed prior to standardization. Unfortunately, no further studies of test fairness or psychometric bias are reported in the test manual.

Validity

Concurrent validity studies with the GAMA were conducted with the Wechsler Adult Intelligence Scale–Revised (WAIS-R; Wechsler, 1981) and the Kaufman Brief Intelligence Test (K-BIT; Kaufman & Kaufman, 1990). A total of 194 individuals between the ages of 25 and 74 years were studied. The GAMA IQ correlated .75 with the WAIS-R FSIQ and .70 with the K-BIT IQ. All three instruments produced mean total test scores that were only slightly discrepant, usually within two standard score points of each other. Similar results are also reported in the GAMA manual for adult ability tests such as the Wonderlic Personnel Test and the Shipley Institute of Living Scale.

Several special population studies are reported in the GAMA Manual. These studies include separate samples of adults with learning disabilities ($n = 34$), traumatic brain injury ($n = 50$), mental retardation ($n = 41$), and deafness ($n = 49$), as well as those who are residing in nursing homes ($n = 43$). Each of these studies provided reasonable evidence for the criterion-related validity of the GAMA, with moderate level correlations and comparable total test scores between the GAMA and the WAIS-R or K-BIT.

See Rapid Reference 2.8 for summary information about the GAMA.

NAGLIERI NONVERBAL ABILITY TEST (NNAT)

The Naglieri Nonverbal Ability Test (NNAT; Naglieri, 1997) is a large scale, group-administered, matrix reasoning test intended for children from kindergarten through grade 12. It is available in seven levels, each with 38 items, specifically normed for appropriate grade levels as well as for fall and spring testing. The NNAT can typically be administered in 30 to 45 minutes. Intended to measure general reasoning ability, the NNAT includes cluster scores for four types of items which are derived from studies of other matrix reasoning

≡ Rapid Reference 2.8

General Ability Measure for Adults (GAMA)

Authors: J. A. Naglieri and A. N. Bardos

Publication date: 1997

What the test measures: General ability, reasoning, and logic

Age range: 18 and older

Administration format: Group or individual

Administration time: 25 minutes

Qualifications of examiners: Interpretation should be conducted by individuals with formal training in assessment (e.g., graduate-level coursework); administration and scoring may be conducted by individuals with less training if they are properly supervised

Publisher: National Computer Systems (NCS)

tasks, constructed according to a specific methodology, and thought to require the use of distinct cognitive abilities.

The NNAT is a revision and extension of the Matrix Analogies Test–Short Form and –Expanded Form (Naglieri, 1985a, 1985b), which employ the same four matrices-based item types (i.e., Pattern Completion, Reasoning by Analogy, Serial Reasoning, and Spatial Reasoning) as well as similar administration procedures (i.e., brief verbal directions). Like the MAT-SF and MAT-EF, the NNAT presents matrices using yellow, blue, and white figural stimuli to minimize the effects of impaired color vision on test performance. The NNAT and the MAT were also designed to assess performance that is not dependent upon stores of acquired knowledge. All of the knowledge needed to solve each item is presented in the item, and factual knowledge, vocabulary, mathematics, and reading skills are not prerequisites for solving NNAT items.

Administration

The NNAT requires about 45 minutes to administer. Approximately 10 minutes are required to complete identification information on the answer document; about 5 minutes are required for verbal instructions and completion of the practice samples. Precisely 30 minutes are allocated for the actual 38 items

≡ Rapid Reference 2.9

NNAT Levels, Recommended Grades, and Normed Grades

Level	Recommended Grades	Ages
A	K	5, 6
B	1	6, 7
C	2	7, 8
D	3, 4	8, 9, 10
E	5, 6	10, 11, 12
F	7, 8, 9	12, 13, 14, 15
G	10, 11, 12	15, 16, 17, 18

that appear at every level. One proctor is recommended for every 25 students.

Students must be able to complete standard, machine-scorable answer documents for this test, including completion of the response circles with a number 2 soft-lead pencil.

The directions for administration appear in English and Spanish and can be given in approximately five minutes. They ask the examinee to identify the answer that will "finish the puzzle" in which there is a piece missing. There are two sample items at each of the seven levels, and correct answers are provided for these to ensure that the examinee understands the task. The levels recommended for students at various grade levels and ages appear in Rapid Reference 2.9.

Scoring and Interpretation

The NNAT is typically machine scored. Students in kindergarten through grade three complete the test in machine-scorable test booklets. Students in grades 4–12 use separate answer documents. Hand-scoring keys are also available.

The NNAT yields a Nonverbal Ability Index (NAI) expressed in standard scores (M = 100, SD = 15), age- and grade-based percentile ranks, stanines, and NCEs; two to four raw cluster scores; and age equivalent scores. The NAI is conceptualized as constituting a measure of overall general ability, rather than specific abilities. According to the technical manual, the NAI is a reliable predictor of a student's academic success.

The NNAT also includes up to four cluster scores, based upon performance on items of four types: Pattern Completion (PC), Reasoning by Analogy (RA), Serial Reasoning (SR), and Spatial Visualization (SV). These cluster scores represent slightly different ways of measuring general ability, based upon prior research.

Pattern Completion (PC). Items in this cluster consist of visual patterns from which a part is missing. The examinee must recognize which of four or five choices contains the same pattern or is continuous with the spatial orientation of the lines in the pattern around the missing part. Pattern completion items tend to appear at the earlier NNAT levels because they involve recognition of visual patterns rather than higher order reasoning or visualization abilities.

Reasoning by Analogy (RA). Items in this cluster require the examinee to recognize a logical relationship between several geometric shapes, based upon the changes in an object across rows and down columns. These items require careful attention to detail and simultaneous processing of multiple features that may be changing in tandem. Reasoning by analogy items tend to span the entire grade range and increase in difficulty by increasing the number of dimensions that are changing in the matrix. For example, a sample item may be verbally mediated as *A white square is to a shaded square as a white circle is to a . . . ?*

Serial Reasoning (SR). Items in this cluster require the examinee to identify a sequential pattern occurring across rows and down columns. Serial Reasoning items tend to span all but the youngest grade range and become more difficult when more than one series is included in the matrix. A progression such as circle–square–triangle is an example of a sequence occurring on an SR item.

Spatial Visualization (SV). Items in this cluster require the examinee to recognize how two or more designs would look if combined or transformed in some systematic manner (e.g., rotated). An example of an SV item is to decide what a design would look like if a circle and triangle were combined. In some cases, designs in a row or column must be added to deduce the correct solution. SV items rank among the most difficult items in the NNAT.

The four clusters are represented by raw scores and do not all appear at every grade level because of their varying levels of difficulty. Rapid Reference 2.10 describes the NNAT clusters that appear at respective testing levels.

≡Rapid Reference 2.10

NNAT Levels and Cluster Content

Level	PC	RA	SR	SV
A	√	√	—	—
B	√	√	√	—
C	√	√	√	√
D	√	√	√	√
E	√	√	√	√
F	—	√	√	√
G	—	√	√	√

Note. PC = Pattern Completion; RA = Reasoning by Analogy; SR = Serial Reasoning; SV = Spatial Visualization.

Strengths and Weaknesses

In this section, several of NNAT's strengths and weaknesses are described. Strengths and weaknesses are also summarized in Rapid Reference 2.11. In brief, the NNAT is well designed for large-scale assessment, and the NNAT's large standardization sample represents a strength unmatched by any other nonverbal test. Its weaknesses include the absence of validity data in the technical manual and its mixture of item types, which sometimes yields extremely low reliabilities for cluster scores.

Ease of Use

Intended for large-scale assessments, NNAT is administered in groups in a single sitting that should require no longer than approximately 45 minutes. It

≡Rapid Reference 2.11

NNAT Strengths and Weaknesses

Strengths	Weaknesses
• Optimal for large-scale assessment • Largest standardization sample for any of the unidimensional nonverbal tests • Brief and easy to administer • English and Spanish directions • Impressive evidence of test fairness	• Absence of validity data reported in test manual • Absence of empirical support for differentiation among four item types • Insufficient balance of item types in clusters at various levels • Highly variable reliabilities for clusters, rendering some unsuitable for interpretation

is typically very easy to administer, requiring only a proctor to read instructions. For large-scale assessments, the NNAT's machine-scoring options and computerized printout make this test perhaps the easiest of nonverbal procedures to administer.

The NNAT is also relatively straightforward for student examinees, although some preschool children may not fully understand the concepts involved in answering the matrices, requiring further explanation.

Selected Technical Features

The NNAT was normed on a very large sample of 89,600 children and adolescents, with geographic region, socioeconomic status, urban/rural setting, ethnicity, and type of school attended as stratifying variables. The norms are weighted according to census proportions and are based upon samples collected in the fall of 1995 ($n = 22,600$) and spring of 1996 ($n = 67,000$). The NNAT was concurrently normed with two group-administered achievement tests, the Stanford Achievement Test Series–Ninth Edition (SAT-9; Harcourt Brace Educational Measurement, 1996) and Aprenda: La prueba de logros en español, Segunda Edición (Aprenda-2; Harcourt Brace Educational Measurement, 1997). This sample represents the largest available for any of the nonverbal cognitive ability tests listed in this chapter.

Based on the Kuder-Richardson Formula #20 reliability coefficients, the NNAT shows evidence of high total test internal score consistency, with reliability coefficients ranging from .83 to .93 by grade (median across all levels is .87) and .81 to .88 by age across the seven levels. The cluster scores, which are based on as few as two items at some levels (e.g., Pattern Completion at Level F) and as many as 30 items at other levels (e.g., Pattern Completion at Level A), vary widely in internal consistency, ranging from .23 to .89. Accordingly, considerable caution should be used in the interpretation of cluster scores.

Fairness

Studies of test bias and fairness are described but not fully reported in the *Technical Manual.* Items were screened with the Mantel-Haenszel procedures for psychometric bias prior to their selection for the final forms of NNAT. These procedures

DON'T FORGET

The NNAT cluster scores may consist of as few as two items at some levels, rendering them unreliable. Interpret only clusters that are based on 15 items or more.

examine differential item functioning between reference (majority) and focal (minority) groups, after matching the groups on ability level. Comparisons were made between males and females, Whites and African Americans, and Whites and Hispanics. Items showing evidence of potential bias using this criterion were removed from the test prior to standardization.

Additional investigations of test fairness with the NNAT are reported by Naglieri and Ronning (in press). They examined differences between three demographically matched samples of white and African American students (n = 2,306 in each group), white and Hispanic students (n = 1,176 in each group), and white and Asian students (n = 466 in each group). Groups were selected from the larger standardization sample and matched according to geographic region, socioeconomic status, ethnicity, and type of school setting (public or private). Effect size differences were reported to be small (d-ratio = .25) for the white and African American samples and small (d-ratio = .17) for the white and Hispanic samples. Effect size differences (d-ratio = .02) were negligible for the white and Asian samples. Accordingly, the NNAT shows small group mean score differences when selected racial and ethnic groups are compared.

Naglieri and Ronning (in press) also report correlations for the same racial and ethnic groups between NNAT performance and performance on Stanford Achievement Tests reading and mathematics tests. Results show that minority groups typically have ability–achievement correlations that are at least as high as those found for the white samples, with no statistically significant differences with a single exception. When the correlations are compared for white and African American samples, the NNAT was found to be a better predictor of reading for African Americans than for white children. Overall, the correlations for the K-12 groups of white/African American, white/Hispanic, and White/Asian varied from a low of .46 to a high of .68 (median = .68), indicating a moderate relationship between the NNAT and achievement in reading and mathematics for the various groups. These results suggest that the NNAT shows fairly comparable prediction of achievement across racial and ethnic groups.

Validity

Few validity studies are reported in the *Technical Manual,* and no convergent validity studies are reported with group-administered or individually-administered measures of cognitive ability or intelligence. Likewise, no special

≡*Rapid Reference 2.12*

Naglieri Nonverbal Ability Test (NNAT)

Authors: Jack A. Naglieri

Publication date: 1997

What the test measures: General nonverbal ability, Pattern Completion, Reasoning by Analogy, Serial Reasoning, and Spatial Visualization

Grade range: K–12

Administration format: Group or individual

Administration time: 35–45 minutes

Qualifications of examiners: Master's level degree in Psychology or Education or the equivalent in a related field, with relevant training in assessment

Publisher: Harcourt Brace Educational Measurement

population studies are reported in the *Technical Manual*. The only studies reported show that the NNAT demonstrates strong correlations with academic achievement, correlating .63, .54, and .64 with SAT-9 total test, reading, and mathematics scores, respectively.

Rapid Reference 2.12 includes general information about the NNAT.

RAVEN'S PROGRESSIVE MATRICES (RPM)

Raven's Progressive Matrices (RPM; Raven, Raven, & Court, 1998) is not a single test but rather a family of matrix reasoning tests. The tests date back to 1938 and include six major versions:

Coloured Progressive Matrices (Classic CPM, or CPM-C). Last revised in 1956, the Classic CPM consists of 36 items presented in color and is intended for use with young children and older individuals, as well as other low ability groups. Norms are available for children ages 5 through 11 and for older adults age 60 and above.

Coloured Progressive Matrices Parallel Version (Parallel CPM, or CPM-P). An equivalent form to the Classic CPM, the Parallel CPM was introduced in 1998 to match the Coloured Progressive Matrices on an item-by-item basis in terms of problem logic, difficulty level, and total score. The Parallel CPM and the Classic CPM may be used interchangeably.

Standard Progressive Matrices (Classic SPM, or SPM-C). Last revised in 1956, the Classic SPM consists of 60 items presented in black and white and is intended to cover a wide range of mental abilities. Norms are available for ages 6 through 68 years or older.

Standard Progressive Matrices Parallel Version (Parallel SPM, or SPM-P). An equivalent form to the Classic SPM, the Parallel SPM was introduced in 1998 to match the Classic SPM on an item-by-item basis in terms of problem solving strategy requirements, item difficulty level, and total score. The Parallel SPM and the Classic SPM may be used interchangeably.

Standard Progressive Matrices Plus (SPM Plus). The SPM Plus is a 60-item test introduced in 1998 to raise the ceiling of the Classic SPM among high ability adolescents and young adults and to restore the test's discriminability among high ability examinees. The SPM Plus eliminated items of intermediate difficulty from the Classic SPM and added more difficult items. The SPM Plus is not interchangeable with the Classic SPM or the Parallel SPM; norms for the Classic SPM may only be used by converting SPM Plus scores to SPM scores (see Rapid Reference 2.14).

Advanced Progressive Matrices (APM, Sets I and II). The APM was last revised in 1962 and consists of two parts: Set I consists of 12 items that may be used as a screening test or practice test, and Set II consists of 36 items that are intended to differentiate individuals of superior intellectual ability. New norms for the APM were published in 1998.

Raven's Progressive Matrices are intended to measure the eductive component of *g* as defined in Spearman's theory of cognitive ability. Eductive ability is defined as the ability to forge new insights, the ability to discern meaning in confusion, the ability to perceive, and the ability to identify relationships. The essential feature of eduction is the ability to generate new, largely nonverbal concepts which make it possible to think clearly. According to the authors (Raven, Raven, & Court, 1998), it is not appropriate to describe the RPM as a measure of general intelligence, ability, or problem solving ability. Moreover, the authors conceptualize the progressive matrices as "unidimensional" in the sense that the tests measure the capacity to engage in intellectual processes that are built one upon another in such a way that people cannot engage in the

> **DON'T FORGET**
>
> Use the CPM with young children and older adults. Use the SPM with most adolescents and adults, and use the APM with intellectually gifted adolescents and adults.

higher order processes unless they have mastered the more basic ones.

In a widely cited investigation of the RPM among young adults, Carpenter, Just, & Shell (1990) developed a detailed theoretical computational model of the processes used in solving the progressive matrices. They concluded, "The processes that distinguish among individuals are primarily the ability to induce abstract relations and the ability to dynamically manage a large set of problem-solving goals in working memory" (p. 404).

Raven's Progressive Matrices are probably the most well known and well researched of nonverbal measures (e.g., Jensen, 1980), having appeared in over 1500 published studies as of the year 2000. The Standard Progressive Matrices were originally developed in the 1930s and initially published in 1938. Normative studies and a linkage to a measure of word knowledge—the Mill Hill Vocabulary Scale—followed during World War II. A modification of the Standard Progressive Matrices was published in 1947, and the CPM and APM were developed. In 1956 the SPM items were resequenced and the CPM and APM were also revised. In the 1980s, item response theory has been used to enhance the comparability and raw score conversions (see Styles & Andrich, 1993) between various versions, for example, between the CPM and SPM, and between the SPM and APM. In 1998, several new versions of the progressive matrices were introduced, including the Parallel SPM, the SPM Plus, and the Parallel CPM. The SPM Plus was introduced to raise the ceiling of the SPM among adolescents and young adults.

Administration

Raven's Progressive Matrices may be administered individually or in groups. Administration directions are verbal and require about 5 to 10 minutes. A proctor for every 10 to 15 examinees is recommended for group testing. Group testing is not recommended for most children under the age of six or seven; an individual testing format is preferable.

Standard administration procedures are relatively simple but have a distinctly British quality to the choice of words: "The top part . . . is a pattern with a bit cut out of it. Look at the pattern, think what the piece needed to complete the pattern correctly both along and down must be like. Then find the right piece out of the six bits shown below" (p. SPM49).

The SPM may also be administered without spoken instructions for examinees who are not proficient in English or for those who are deaf. The examiner points to the main figure and then to the gap in it. He or she then teaches the task by pointing to each of the multiple choice options, either shaking (or nodding) his or her head depending on whether the option is the correct response.

In general, all of the Progressive Matrices may be administered in less than an hour. Although a common practice, the authors of the RPM recommend against timing, noting that it emphasizes speed and efficiency and "seriously discriminates against those who work more slowly and carefully" (p. SPM6). The Coloured Progressive Matrices require up to about 30 minutes to administer; the Standard Progressive Matrices require up to about 45 minutes to administer; and the Advanced Progressive Matrices require up to about an hour to administer.

Several computerized versions of the RPM have been developed. Raven, Raven, and Court (1998) report equivalence between paper-and-pencil versions of the test and computerized versions. Self-scoring test forms are also available.

Scoring and Interpretation

All answers on Raven's Progressive Matrices are multiple choice. Individual administration requires the examiner to record the answer corresponding to the multiple choice selection made by the examinee. Response may be scored in multiple ways, including the use of a scoring key that must be correctly aligned next to the appropriate column and row. One point is awarded for each correct response. The total score is the total number correct.

Raw scores may be converted from CPM to and from Classic SPM or Parallel SPM, from Classic SPM or Parallel SPM to and from SPM Plus, or from Classic or Parallel SPM to APM and back, using Tables SPM3 to SPM6 (Raven, Raven, & Court, 1998, Section 3). The most common conversions, those between the Coloured Progressive Matrices and the Standard Progressive Matrices, appear in Rapid Reference 2.13. Conversions from the SPM Plus to the SPM are also provided in Rapid Reference 2.14.

Examiners must select from numerous normative choices, most of which have some limitations which are further discussed below.

Raven's Progressive Matrices yield age-based percentile ranks and gross descriptive categories (intellectually superior, definitely above the average, intellectually average, and definitely below the average).

≡Rapid Reference 2.13

Raw Score Conversions between the Standard Progressive Matrices and Coloured Progressive Matrices

Raw Scores

CPM	SPM	CPM	SPM	CPM	SPM
0	0	13	12	26	29
1	1	14	13	27	30
2	2	15	14	28	32
3	3	16	15	29	35
4	4	17	16	30	36
5	5	18	17	31	39
6	6	19	19	32	41
7	7	20	20	33	44
8	8	21	21	34	48
9	9	22	22	35	52
10	9	23	24	36	57
11	10	24	26		
12	11	25	27		

Rapid Reference 2.14

Raw Score Conversions between the Standard Progressive Matrices Plus and the Classic/Parallel Standard Progressive Matrices

Raw Scores

SPM Plus	SPM-C or SPM-P	SPM Plus	SPM-C or SPM-P
1	1, 2	28	38
2	3	29	39
3	4	30	40
4	5, 6	31	41, 42
5	7	32	43
6	8	33	44
7	9	34	45
8	10	35	46
9	11, 12	36	47
10	13	37	48
11	14	38	49
12	15, 16	39	50
13	17	40, 41	51
14	18	42	52
15	19	43, 44	53
16	20, 21	45	54
17	22	46, 47	55
18	23, 24	48, 49	56
19	25	50, 51	57
20	26, 27	52, 53, 54	58
21	28	55	59
22	29, 30	56	
23	31	57	
24	32	58	
25	33, 34	59	
26	35	60	
27	36, 37		

The test is generally interpreted at the total score level, although numerous attempts have been made to interpret the matrices according to item set, errors, factors, content of individual items, and time to completion. Analysis of errors has been proposed as a supplementary approach to interpretation for the CPM and the APM, although

> # DON'T FORGET
> ....
> Raw scores on different versions of the Raven's Progressive Matrices may be converted to expected raw scores on other versions for the purpose of making comparisons between tests: CPM to SPM and back, SPM to SPM Plus and back, and SPM to APM and back.

Raven, Raven, and Court (1998) suggest that "information on the nature of the errors people make usually adds little to that provided by their total score" (p. CPM4).

Strengths and Weaknesses

With its large body of research, Raven's Progressive Matrices represent a historic standard among matrices-based unidimensional intelligence tests and are widely regarded as a relatively pure measure of *g,* or general intellectual ability. To the authors' credit, the tests continue to be enhanced with each revision. These efforts have addressed some major psychometric problems, such as inadequate ceiling in the Standard Progressive Matrices. At the same time, the failure to develop nationally representative, demographically stratified norms in the United States continues to render the RPM the only major nonverbal instrument not having adequate U.S. norms. Moreover, the multiplicity of tests (i.e., Classic CPM, Parallel CPM, Classic SPM, Parallel SPM, SPM Plus, and APM Sets I and II) and the need to select an appropriate normative reference group for each test can be challenging and diminish the ease of use. The striking discrepancy between the RPM's remarkable strengths and glaring weaknesses is described in the following sections (see also Rapid Reference 2.15).

Ease of Use

Raven's Progressive Matrices are extremely easy to use, once the decision has been made about which of the test versions to use and which norms to apply. Answering this question, however, is a considerable challenge because the test manuals are somewhat inconsistent. In general, low ability examinees (e.g.,

≡ *Rapid Reference 2.15*

Raven's Progressive Matrices Strengths and Weaknesses

Strengths	Weaknesses
• Easy to administer	• Ambiguity about indications for use of each test
• The most researched of unidimensional nonverbal cognitive tests	• Problems with test ceilings (e.g., SPM) and with the norms on the new test (SPM Plus) developed to solve the ceiling problems
• Availability of different tests and norms for different purposes	
• New tables enhance comparison and interchangeability between tests	• Normative samples are inadequate for United States
• Good convergent validity with other IQ tests	

children between the ages of about 5 and 10 or 11, and older adults showing evidence of cognitive deterioration) may be administered the Coloured Progressive Matrices; most adolescents and low or average functioning adults may be administered the Standard Progressive Matrices; and high ability adolescents and adults should be administered either the SPM Plus or the Advanced Progressive Matrices Sets I and II. Because the SPM Plus does not yet have independent norms, it can only be interpreted by converting its scores to Classic SPM scores (see Rapid Reference 2.14), and this conversion effectively minimizes many of the benefits of its increased ceiling.

Lists of advantages and disadvantages of each version for specific groups and applications are provided in the test manuals, making it difficult for even experienced testers to make some decisions. For example, in discussing high ability adults, the authors note that the SPM's format across item sets allows examinees five successive opportunities to acquire a sense of what is required and to develop an appropriate method of working; that is, they have an opportunity to learn from experience in solving the matrices. Accordingly, the SPM is recommended if the examiner believes that the examinee would benefit from such learning while taking the test. By contrast, the APM offers less opportunity to learn from taking the test itself. Similar discussions are presented regarding timing of the tests, individual or group testing, computerized administration, and other issues. While these discussions empower the examiner to make informed decisions in choosing the right tests and testing conditions, they also introduce an element of ambiguity that negates the simplicity of the progressive matrices. A simpler recommendation might be to select the test that has the most rigorous norms for the intended examinee. An examination of norms, however, reveals further problems with the RPM, as we will now discuss.

Selected Technical Features

The Coloured Progressive Matrices, the Standard Progressive Matrices, and the Advanced Progressive Matrices each offer over 15 independent reference norms for examiners to utilize. These norms were collected internationally between the 1970s and the 1990s, among samples widely varying in quality. The availability of these norms provides test users with a wide array of options but insufficient information to make informed decisions about the representativeness of each sample. Moreover, virtually none of the norms approach the careful sampling utilized by the other nonverbal tests described in this book.

For example, the most recent standardization in the United States occurred in 1993 for the APM and the SPM. The sample consisted of 625 adults over the age of 17 who resided in Des Moines, Iowa. A random sampling within census blocks (geographic units that are representative of the population to be studied in terms of age, ethnicity, and socioeconomic status) was undertaken in Des Moines, using the logic that Des Moines is one of four U.S. cities having demographic characteristics that approximate those of the United States as a whole. Accordingly, the results from the standardization in Des Moines are considered by the test authors to be representative of the United States as a whole.

The sophistication of this sampling approach is undermined by the results. Only 7% of the population of Des Moines is African American, whereas the figure for the United States as a whole is at least 12%, suggesting that at least one minority group was significantly underrepresented in the sample. The failure to report a detailed description of the normative sample, and the degree to which it resembles the U.S. population as a whole, does not meet available reporting standards for psychological and educational tests. Finally, the authors acknowledge that "these Des Moines norms are probably above those which would have been obtained had a random sample of the entire U.S. population been tested" (p. SPM14). Many of the norms appearing throughout the Progressive Matrices have this same quality—of being ambitious in their scope but not representative of their populations.

Norms for the RPM may also be criticized in some cases for their obsolescence. The RPM have been the primary tests used to demonstrate the Flynn effect, that is, the phenomenon that IQs have been rising in developed countries for at least three generations at a rate of approximately three IQ points per decade, or about one standard deviation per generation. For example, on the Classic SPM, people born in 1877 and tested in 1942 averaged 24 raw score points on the SPM, while people born in 1967 and measured in 1992 averaged 54 raw score points. Both were said to have an IQ of 100 in the respective years on their evaluations. These improvements in the test-based intelligence of the general population are a primary reason why Raven, Raven, and Court (1998) created the SPM Plus to raise the ceiling of the SPM. They also constitute a well-established reason to avoid the use of norms that date back more than a decade or so, as many of the reported Raven's norms do.

Reliability coefficients for the RPM tend to meet existing standards, and results from multiple studies described in the manuals are summarized here. For the Classic CPM, investigations of more than 1500 young children have yielded a split-half reliability coefficient of .90, with no differences by ethnicity or sex. The majority of studies with the Classic SPM yield a split-half reliability coefficient exceeding .90, with a modal value of .91. Finally, somewhat reduced reliability results are evident for the APM, which is intended for high ability populations. The APM Set I (a 12-item set) is reported to have a split-half reliability coefficient of .73, whereas the longer Set II has a split-half reliability coefficient between .83 and .87.

Test-retest stability coefficients for the Classic CPM tend to range from .81 to .95 over a test-retest interval of 10 days to one month. Stability coefficients for the Classic SPM tend to be about .90 over short-term intervals (e.g., one week), falling to .80 at longer intervals (e.g., one to three months). On the APM, stability coefficients of .80 to .91 have been reported for adolescents and adults.

Examination of the ceilings and floors of the RPM suggests some difficulties, which the authors have begun to address. The test manuals fail to report what percentage of children can correctly complete at least one item (one indication of *floor*, or the lowest ages or ability levels at which the test retains discriminability) and what percentage of individuals correctly respond to every item (an indication of *ceiling,* or the highest ages or ability levels at which the test retains discriminability). The manuals do, however, provide raw scores corresponding to the 5th and 95th percentile ranks. On the CPM, 5½-year-old children who correctly answer 8 out of the 36 items rank at the 5th percentile, suggesting that this test probably has an adequate floor at ages five and six. By about age 9, a nearly perfect score (35 correct out of 36 items) is obtained by the upper five percent of the normative sample, suggesting that a ceiling has probably been reached. At this point, the SPM would be appropriate for use. The SPM was intended to cover a wide range of mental ability for adolescents and adults, but a significant ceiling effect has been demonstrated among older adolescents and young adults. According to available norms, a full 5% of adolescents and adults will correctly answer 59 out of the 60 items by the age of 18, indicating that the SPM cannot discriminate among intellectually gifted adults who rank in the top 2 percent (+2 SD) of the normative sample. This limited ceiling was the impetus for the creation of the SPM Plus, which extends the range of SPM item difficulties to discriminate among high ability individuals. Because the SPM Plus has not yet been normed, it should be considered experimental until norms and percentile ranks are available. Accordingly, neither the SPM nor the SPM Plus should be used to identify older adolescents or adults who may be intellectually gifted. The APM is a far more appropriate instrument for such purposes. A score of 33 correct out of 36 items on the APM Set II is ranked at the 97th percentile for young adults, suggesting that there is an improved ceiling on this instrument relative to the SPM, but that the test is unlikely to extend to more than three standard deviations above the normative mean. A time limit is probably necessary to use the APM to assess exceptionally gifted adolescents and adults.

Fairness

As a family of measures usually thought to be culture fair and to have international applications, Raven's Progressive Matrices have provided pioneering methodologies to establish test fairness. At the same time, the instruments continue to yield group mean score differences that have contributed to debates about race and intelligence. For example, Jensen (1980) used the Coloured Progressive Matrices as a standard measure of his Level II ability (i.e., transformation of stimuli through skills such as reasoning and problem solving) to explain what he argued are genuine differences between African Americans and whites that cannot be dismissed as cultural bias.

One approach to demonstrating test fairness using item response theory is to compare the item difficulty calibrations across independent racial and ethnic groups. With the Standard Progressive Matrices, correlations between item difficulties ranged from .97 to .99 in eight separate socioeconomic groups, based on the 1979 British standardization. In the U.S. standardization, the correlations between item difficulties for African American, white, Hispanic, Asian, and Navajo groups ranged from .97 to 1.00, demonstrating that the test has similar psychometric properties across these groups. Jensen (1980) has presented similar findings for the Coloured Progressive Matrices.

The SPM have also been demonstrated to have comparable validity in predicting achievement across racial and ethnic groups in the United States. While group mean scores tend to be different, the regression lines of the SPM on achievement are parallel across racial and ethnic groups in studies by Jensen (1980).

In a pioneering study, Saccuzzo and Johnson (1995) examined a proportionate representation model of test bias with a total of 26,300 males and females from eight different racial and ethnic backgrounds over a nine-year period. The Wechsler intelligence scales and the SPM were shown to have comparable predictive validity and no evidence of differential validity, although significant differences were found as a function of ethnic background between those who were referred for gifted and talented placement and those who scored in the 98th percentile on either test. Moreover, use of the SPM appears to have resulted in increased (but not proportionate) representation of minority students certified as gifted. The authors consider this conclusion to be tentative, however, because of changes in the referral process and samples assessed.

Validity

A considerable amount of research is available to demonstrate the validity of the Raven's Progressive Matrices. Much of it involves criterion-related concurrent validity studies, such as correlations with other measures of g or general intellectual ability, but many additional predictive validity, factor analytic, and special population investigations have also been conducted. This research is adequately summarized in the test manuals and will only briefly be reiterated here.

Investigations relating the Coloured Progressive Matrices to other intelligence tests generally show moderately high correlations, ranging from .43 to .96 with the Stanford-Binet and the Wechsler intelligence scales but generally clustering at about .60 to .70, showing higher correlations with the Wechsler performance scales than verbal scales. Correlations between the Standard Progressive Matrices and the Stanford-Binet and Wechsler intelligence scales generally range from .54 to .86, again showing higher correlations with performance than verbal scales. Correlations between the Advanced Progressive Matrices and the Wechsler scales have been reported in the .70s. These studies have been conducted on a variety of samples, often without corrections for restriction or expansion of range. However, the preponderance of the investigations provides support for conceptualizing the Raven's Progressive Matrices as a good measure of g.

Predictive validity has been demonstrated to be generally impressive, albeit again with significant variability across studies. Raven's Progressive Matrices have been shown to have moderately high correlations with such external criterion variables as school grades, examination results, teacher ratings, educational and occupational attainment by adults, and the level of job people attain and retain.

In factor analytic investigations across multiple cognitive and intellectual tests, the RPM have been associated with a variety of overlapping cognitive abilities, including simultaneous processing, fluid intelligence, visuospatial ability, and inductive reasoning. Raven, Raven, and Court (1998) conclude, "The evidence from factor-analytic research suggests, then, that while SPM is a relatively good measure of general intellectual ability it is not a pure g estimate" (p. SPM34).

Among special populations, scores on the progressive matrices have been shown to decline progressively with degenerative and dementing disorders. Attempts to relate the lateralization of brain injury to RPM performance have yielded equivocal results, with some investigations showing that examinees with left cerebral hemisphere damage perform worse than those with right cerebral hemisphere damage, while others show the converse. The only conclusion that may be drawn is that performance on the progressive matrices is

======*Rapid Reference 2.16*

Raven's Progressive Matrices (RPM)

Authors: J. Raven, J. C. Raven, and J. H. Court

Publication date: 1956, 1962, and 1998 for the tests; 1998 for the newest revisions of the test manuals

What the test measures: Eductive ability

Age range: 5 through adulthood

Administration format: Group or individual

Administration time: Untimed; generally less than 60 minutes

Qualifications of examiners: Master's level degree in Psychology or Education or the equivalent in a related field with relevant training in assessment

Publisher: Oxford Psychologists Press

---

dependent upon numerous cognitive processes mediated by both cerebral hemispheres.

Rapid Reference 2.16 contains overview information about Raven's Progressive Matrices.

TEST OF NONVERBAL INTELLIGENCE (TONI-III)

The Test of Nonverbal Intelligence–Third Edition (TONI-III; Brown, Sherbenou, & Johnsen, 1997) is an individually-administered, matrix-formatted measure of "abstract/figural problem solving" normed for use with individuals between the ages of 6 years and 89 years. Requiring about 15 to 20 minutes to administer, the test is available in two parallel forms (A and B) and is administered with pantomimed and gestural instructions that are completely nonverbal and language free. Intended to measure abstract reasoning and problem solving, the TONI-III is thought to provide an estimate of fluid intelligence and general intellectual ability. Performance on the TONI-III was intended to be minimally influenced by the requirements of language and culture.

The TONI-III is a revision of the test first published in 1982 and revised in 1990. Relative to prior editions, the newest edition has been trimmed by nearly one-fifth to 45 items, and it features new stimuli drawings. The TONI-III includes a new and expanded normative base of 3,451 children, adolescents, and adults, as well as additional studies of validity and fairness.

Administration

The TONI-III is administered through pantomimed instructions with no overt language. The Picture Book is placed between the examiner and examinee. The examinee is required to indicate which of four to six multiple choice options best completes a figural matrix. The examinee responds gesturally, usually by pointing, although the test can be adapted for individuals with severe handicapping conditions so as to permit eye blinks, head sticks, light beams, or other mechanisms of response.

A series of five training items, for which responses are not recorded or scored, are then administered to ensure that the examinee understands task expectations. The examiner points to the empty box in the stimulus portion of the item at the top of the page, points to and runs a finger across the response choices at the bottom of the page, points to the empty square again, and looks questioningly at the examinee. The examiner subsequently points to incorrect responses, shaking his or her head "No," subsequently pointing to a correct response while shaking his or her head "Yes." The practice items may be repeated if necessary.

The test is untimed, and administration continues until a ceiling of three incorrect responses in five consecutive items is reached.

Scoring

The TONI-III Record Form is easy to use. The examiner records an "X" over the number corresponding to the choice made by the examinee. The correct answer is printed in boldface type inside a circle. A score of 1 is awarded to every correct response, and 0 to every incorrect response. The Total Raw Score is the number of correct responses between Item 1 and the ceiling item (or the end of the test, if a ceiling is not reached). The Total Raw Score may be converted to a TONI-III Quotient (M = 100, SD = 15), percentile ranks, descriptive classifications, and age-equivalent scores.

Interpretation

The TONI-III Quotient is a composite score measuring general intelligence, particularly abstract reasoning, problem solving, and other aspects of fluid intelligence. It spans ability levels ranging from Very Poor to Very Superior. The principal value of the TONI-III is as a screener or brief estimate of cognitive ability, and its authors caution against overgeneralization of TONI-III results: "We recognize that it will not usually be a reasonable substitute for broad-based tests of intelligence or aptitude" (Brown, Sherbenou, & Johnsen, 1997, p. 70).

The TONI-III requires the examinee to apply a variety of complex reasoning strategies to abstract/figural content. Stimuli in the TONI-III vary according to the following constituent characteristics: shape, position, direction, rotation, contiguity, shading, size, and movement. Unfortunately, the TONI-III does not offer any scoring methodology by which strategies or responses to specific types of problems may be quantified.

Strengths and Weaknesses

In this section, several strengths and weaknesses of the TONI-III are presented. As summarized in Rapid Reference 2.17, strengths of the TONI-III include its ease of use, nonverbal administration, parallel equivalent forms, and evidence of test fairness. Weaknesses include several technical properties that are insufficiently or inappropriately reported in an otherwise thoughtful and thorough test manual.

⩵Rapid Reference 2.17

TONI-III Strengths and Weaknesses

Strengths	Weaknesses
• Brief and easy to use	• Insufficient information provided to evaluate representativeness of normative sample
• 100% nonverbal administration	
• Two parallel forms	• Inappropriate and inflated reporting of test reliabilities
• Good evidence of test fairness	

Ease of Use

The brevity and simplicity of the TONI-III represents a major strength. It requires no language and can be taught with simple gestures. It can be administered in 15 to 20 minutes, and it has two parallel forms to track changes in cognitive functioning across serial evaluations. Its multiple choice format minimizes scoring errors. The TONI-III represents a very easy screener to administer and score.

Selected Technical Features

The technical features of the TONI-III appear to meet conventional psychometric standards, although the failure to report some information (i.e., representativeness of the normative sample across races and ethnicities according to socioeconomic stratifications) and the inclusion of spurious methodologies to inflate reliabilities detracts from the confidence users can place in this test.

The TONI-III was normed in 1995–1996 on a sample of 3,451 individuals between the ages of 6 and 89 in four geographic regions. The sample was stratified by gender, race, urban/rural residence, ethnicity, family income, parent or adult educational attainment, and disability. The sample appears to be adequately representative of the U.S. population, although no information is presented in the manual describing proportionate representation of groups according to socioeconomic stratification variables. A common sampling limitation of standardized tests includes a failure to balance varying socioeconomic status across racial and ethnic groups, instead drawing the entire low income sample from certain races and ethnicities.

Internal consistency indices of score reliability appear to meet technical standards of adequacy. Across 20 age groups, the average coefficient alpha for the total score is .93 for Form A and .93 for Form B. Reliabilities are similarly high for subsets of the normative sample, including male, female, African American, Hispanic, deaf, gifted, and learning disabled individuals. Test-retest score reliability was assessed through an investigation of examinees who were adolescents and adults, with an average test-retest interval of one week. Overall, the test-retest coefficients were greater than .90 for both forms.

In spite of the TONI-III's more than adequate level of score reliability, the authors of the TONI-III also present interscorer reliability calculations (calculated at .99, and unusual for multiple choice tests in which *no* examiner judgment is required to score items) and *then* average reliabilities for internal consistency, test-retest stability, and interscorer agreement to obtain a spuriously high (.96) estimate of measurement precision. The inclusion of this composite reliability is ill-advised and misleading.

Equivalency between Forms A and B is demonstrated through concurrent administration of both forms in a single testing session to the entire normative sample. The mean difference between the two forms is 0.5 raw score points, and the two forms correlate at .84 and range from .79 to .95. The manual does not document whether the parallel forms were administered in counterbalanced order.

Validity

The TONI-III has been studied in three criterion-related concurrent validity studies. These investigations suggest that the TONI-III Quotient is highly correlated with other unidimensional tests and with the WAIS-R Full Scale IQ, but only at moderate levels with the WISC-III Full Scale IQ. The TONI-III Quotient is correlated more highly with Performance IQ than Verbal IQ, but only for the WAIS-R and not for the WISC-III. These studies are generally commensurate with results of previous studies, but salient information such as standard deviations that may be used to correct the correlations are not reported. Nonetheless, these findings are briefly detailed below.

In a sample of 550 adults between the ages of 19 and 50, the TONI-III Quotient for Forms A and B correlated respectively at .76 and .74 with the CTONI Nonverbal IQ, .74 and .72 with the Pictorial Nonverbal IQ, and .64 and .64 with the Geometric Nonverbal IQ. In a sample of 34 children diagnosed with learning disabilities, ranging in age from 7 years to 17 years, the TONI-III Quotient for Forms A and B correlated respectively at .63 and .63 with the WISC-III Full Scale IQ, .59 and .53 with the Verbal IQ, and .56 and .58 with the Performance IQ. Finally, in a sample of 19 adolescents diagnosed with learning disabilities, ranging in age from 16 years to 19 years, the TONI-III Quotient for Forms A and B correlated respectively at .73 and .71 with the WAIS-R Full Scale IQ, .57 and .51 with the Verbal IQ, and .75 and .76 with the Performance IQ.

Investigations exploring the relationship between the TONI-III Quotient and tests of achievement suggest moderate to high correlations, especially in areas of academic skill that are more fluid and less dependent on stores of acquired knowledge. In these studies, a small sample of 20 students diagnosed with learning disabilities was administered the TONI-III and two achievement tests. The TONI-III Quotient for Forms A and B correlated respectively at .59 and .58 with the Diagnostic Achievement Battery (DAB-2) Writing Comprehension, .73 and .71 with the Woodcock-Johnson Psycho-Educational Battery–Revised (WJ-R) Broad Reading, .76 and .74 with the WJ-R Broad Mathematics, .56 and .55 with WJ-R Broad Knowledge, and .76 and .70 with WJ-R Skills.

Special population studies with the TONI-III suggest that the test may be useful in identifying individuals with mental retardation (Mean TONI-III Quotient = 71; $n = 27$) but somewhat less useful with individuals who are intellectually gifted (Mean TONI-III Quotient = 110; $n = 111$). Group mean scores were fully within the average range of expectations for individuals diagnosed with dyslexia ($n = 51$), attention deficit hyperactivity disorder (Mean TONI-III Quotient = 98; $n = 131$), learning disabilities (Mean TONI-III Quotient = 95; $n = 287$), and emotional disturbance (Mean TONI-III Quotient = 94; $n = 55$).

Fairness

The TONI-III utilizes two separate psychometric indices of item bias: comparisons of item characteristic curves and comparisons of item difficulties across seven gender, racial, ethnic, and exceptionality subgroups.

Based upon item response theory (IRT), the authors conducted nonparametric statistical comparison of item characteristic curves (ICCs) using the Standard Index of Bias with the seven subgroups to ensure that the groups have similar curve characteristics. Results show that for each of the seven subgroups, a range of one to five items on each form show statistically significant differences indicating psychometric bias.

Relative item difficulties across seven subgroups were also compared through correlations of Delta scores, yielding correlations of .98 and .99. These findings suggest that item difficulties are comparable across the groups studied.

Separate investigations demonstrate that internal consistency (coefficient alpha) is comparable from the overall standardization sample to subgroups based on gender, race, ethnicity, deafness, and disability.

An overview of the TONI-III appears in Rapid Reference 2.18.

≡Rapid Reference 2./8

Test of Nonverbal Intelligence–Third Edition (TONI-III)

Authors: Linda Brown, Rita J. Sherbenou, and Susan K. Johnsen
Publication date: 1997
What the test measures: Nonverbal reasoning ability
Age range: 6 through 89
Administration format: Individual
Administration time: 15 to 20 minutes
Qualifications of examiners: The TONI-III may be administered by psychologists, psychological associates, educational diagnosticians, teachers, counselors, speech and language therapists, and other qualified professionals who have had formal training in psychological assessment.
Publisher: Pro-Ed

SUMMARY

Chapter Two describes the major unidimensional nonverbal tests of intelligence, including the Beta III, CTONI, GAMA, NNAT, Raven's, and TONI-III. These tests are considered unidimensional primarily because of their relatively limited format. That is, most rely on a single format presentation, either easel-based or booklet. The most common format is based on the matrix analogies design. The tests are probably most commonly used as screening instruments, rather than for diagnostic or decision-making purposes. Also, even though the psychometric properties are impressive for several of these instruments, the depth and breadth of interpretation are limited. In addition, the clinical testing observations are necessarily limited because the tests do not require multiple response modes; that is, typically they require only manipulation of pencil and paper. Their primary strengths are efficiency and ease of administration.

TEST YOURSELF

1. **Which of the following is an advantage of multidimensional nonverbal tests relative to unidimensional tests?**

   (a) Brevity and cost effectiveness

   (b) Ease of administration

   (c) Testing efficiency

   (d) Broad-based assessment

2. **What is one advantage of unidimensional nonverbal tests relative to multidimensional tests?**

   (a) Usually report more validity data

   (b) Can be useful for placement decisions

   (c) Broad-based assessment

   (d) Testing efficiency

3. **Which unidimensional test is not normed for use with adults?**

   (a) Beta III

   (b) Comprehensive Test of Nonverbal Intelligence (CTONI)

   (c) Test of Nonverbal Intelligence (TONI-III)

   (d) Naglieri Nonverbal Ability Test (NNAT)

4. **Which unidimensional test has no verbal instructional set?**

   (a) Beta III

   (b) General Ability Measure for Adults (GAMA)

   (c) Test of Nonverbal Intelligence (TONI-III)

   (d) Raven's Progressive Matrices

5. **Which unidimensional test has a parallel or equivalent form?**

   (a) Beta III

   (b) Comprehensive Test of Nonverbal Intelligence (CTONI)

   (c) General Ability Measure for Adults (GAMA)

   (d) Test of Nonverbal Intelligence (TONI-III)

6. **Which unidimensional test has the largest national normative sample?**

   (a) Comprehensive Test of Nonverbal Intelligence (CTONI)

   (b) General Ability Measure for Adults (GAMA)

   (c) Test of Nonverbal Intelligence (TONI-III)

   (d) Naglieri Nonverbal Ability Test (NNAT)

(continued)

7. **Which unidimensional test may be group-administered?**

   (a) Beta III

   (b) Columbia

   (c) Leiter-R

   (d) Test of Nonverbal Intelligence (TONI-III)

8. **Which unidimensional test has been most thoroughly researched in the professional literature?**

   (a) Beta III

   (b) Comprehensive Test of Nonverbal Intelligence (CTONI)

   (c) General Ability Measure for Adults (GAMA)

   (d) Raven's Progressive Matrices

9. **Which is not a formal definition of eductive ability?**

   (a) Ability to forge new insights

   (b) Ability to discern meaning in confusion

   (c) Ability to perceive

   (d) Ability to plan

10. **Which of the Raven's Progressive Matrices are appropriate for younger children?**

   (a) Classic Coloured Progressive Matrices

   (b) Classic Standard Progressive Matrices

   (c) Standard Progressive Matrices Plus

   (d) Advanced Progressive Matrices

Answers: 1. d; 2. d; 3. d; 4. c; 5. d; 6. d; 7. a; 8. d; 9. d; 10. a

Three

MULTIDIMENSIONAL NONVERBAL INTELLIGENCE TESTS: ADMINISTRATION, SCORING, AND INTERPRETATION OF THE UNIT

There are a number of unidimensional nonverbal tests available to assess intelligence; the six major unidimensional tests are described in Chapter 2. On the other hand, there are only two currently available nonverbal tests that could accurately be described as multidimensional: the Universal Nonverbal Intelligence Test (UNIT; Bracken & McCallum, 1998), published by the Riverside Publishing Company, and the Leiter International Performance Scale–Revised (Leiter-R; Roid & Miller, 1997), published by the Stoelting Company. Multidimensional tests typically consist of several subtests, which in turn combine to yield more global scale scores. Most multidimensional tests of intelligence also yield one global score, often referred to as a "full scale," "general," or "broad" ability measure. Because these tests have multiple components, and because they tend to have good psychometric properties, they are sometimes used to make important educational placement decisions. For example, scores may be used to determine whether examinees are eligible for placement in classes that serve children with learning disabilities or mental retardation. Consequently, multidimensional tests are sometimes referred to as "high stakes" tests.

Multidimensional tests not only yield scores that can be used for eligibility decisions, they also provide information about an examinee's cognitive strengths and weaknesses. The subtest scores may be interpreted normatively (i.e., relative to peers) or ipsatively (i.e., relative to examinee's own mean). There is considerable controversy in the literature regarding the efficacy of subtest interpretation. Some experts argue in favor of using subtest scores as a basis for explaining certain academic problems and for planning subsequent remediational strategies in an aptitude X treatment paradigm (e.g., Kaufman, 1979, 1994; Sattler, 1988). Others oppose specific subtest interpretation, arguing that subtests are psychometrically inadequate (e.g., McDermott, Fantuzzo, & Glutting, 1990). In spite of the controversy, many clinicians find interpretation of subtest profiles helpful, relying on the assumption that scores vary because of systematic and real cognitive abilities, and that these abilities are related to meaningful functioning in the classroom and the workplace.

Two nonverbal intelligence tests are particularly amenable to both normative and ipsative interpretation: the UNIT and the Leiter-R. Both are multidimensional; both yield subtest scores, more global scale scores, and a full scale score. The UNIT was developed more recently, contains fewer subtests, and is less cumbersome to administer and interpret. Consequently, we describe it first.

HISTORY AND DEVELOPMENT OF THE UNIT

Intelligence should not be conceptualized as being either verbal or nonverbal. Rather, there are verbal and nonverbal methods available to assess intelligence. At the most basic level, the UNIT can be conceptualized as a measure of intelligence, conducted nonverbally. Consequently, the UNIT should be considered a nonverbal measure of intelligence, not a measure of nonverbal intelligence. According to many experts (e.g., Carroll, 1993; Jensen, 1980), intelligence consists primarily of a pervasive and fundamental ability, g, which provides a base for the development of somewhat unique specialized skills. Although the UNIT is designed to provide a unique measure of cognitive organization (i.e., symbolic and nonsymbolic content) and function (memory and reasoning), it is first and foremost a strong measure of g, primarily because of the cognitive complexity required by each of the subtests. Even the memory subtests were designed to require considerable cognitive engagement (i.e., multiple salient features to remember).

Specifically, the UNIT is designed to assess functioning according to a two-tier model of intelligence; task completion requires primarily memory or reasoning and one of two organizational strategies (symbolic and nonsymbolic organization; see Bracken & McCallum, 1998). Of the six subtests included on the UNIT, three require memory primarily; these subtests are Object Memory (OM), Spatial Memory (SpaM), and Symbolic Memory (SymM). Similarly, three subtests were developed to assess reasoning primarily; these subtests are Cube Design (CD), Mazes (M), and Analogic Reasoning (AR). Five of the subtests require minor motoric manipulation (i.e., CD, OM, M, SymM, SpaM), and one requires only a pointing response (AR). With two exceptions (CD, M), the subtests that require motoric manipulation can be adapted to allow for a pointing response only, as needed.

As operationalized on the UNIT, symbolic organizational strategies require the use of concrete and abstract symbols to conceptualize the environment; these symbols are typically language related (e.g., words), although symbols may take on any form (e.g., numbers, statistical equations, Rebus characters, flags). Cognitive development enables individuals to internalize symbols as they begin to label, mediate, designate, and over time, make experiences meaningful. Nonsymbolic strategies require the ability to perceive and make meaningful judgments about the physical relationships within our environment; this ability is symbol-free, or relatively so, and is closer to fluid-like intellectual abilities. Nonsymbolic strategies are more likely to require the ability to discern and discriminate abstract geometric patterns, for example.

As implied above, within each of the two fundamental organizational categories (nonsymbolic and symbolic) of the UNIT, problem solution requires one of two types of abilities: memory or reasoning. That is, some of the items require primarily symbolic organization and rely heavily on memory (e.g., those included on the Symbolic Memory subtests). Other items require considerable symbolic organization and reasoning skills, but less memory (e.g., those included on the Analogic Reasoning subtests). Some items seem to require nonsymbolic organizational strategies and memory (e.g., those on the Spatial Memory subtest). Finally, others may require nonsymbolic organization and reasoning and little memory (Cube Design). Consequently, the UNIT assesses four basic cognitive abilities operationalized by the six subtests (see Rapid Reference 3.1).

The rationale for assessing intelligence using the four strategies operationalized by the UNIT is based on several lines of theory and research. For example, Wechsler emphasized the importance of distinguishing between highly symbolic (verbal) versus nonsymbolic (performance) expression in 1939. Jensen (1980) provides the rationale for a two-tiered hierarchical conceptualization of intelligence, consisting of the two subconstructs of memory (Level I) and reasoning (Level II). (It should be noted that many currently available Level I memory tasks are characterized by low g-loadings and are designed to require reproduction or recall of simple content; in contrast, UNIT memory tasks were developed to require more complex memory.) UNIT reasoning tasks were designed to require the ability to comprehend, analyze, and synthesize the organizational aspects of content, concepts and ideas.

≡ Rapid Reference 3. 1

Conceptual Model for the UNIT

	Memory Subtests	Reasoning Subtests
Symbolic Subtests	Symbolic Memory Object Memory	Analogic Reasoning
Nonsymbolic Subtests	Spatial Memory	Cube Design Mazes

The theoretical organization of the UNIT is consistent with a number of newly developed instruments which adopt the Gf-Gc Model of fluid and crystallized abilities, as described by Cattell (1963), Horn (1968), and others (e.g., Woodcock, 1990). Memory and reasoning are two important subconstructs identified in the Gf-Gc Model. In fact, according to an analysis presented by McGrew and Flannagan (1998) in their *Intelligence Test Desk Reference,* UNIT subtests assess a number of the Gf-Gc stratum II and III abilities, as described in Table 3.1.

Table 3.1 UNIT Gc-Gf Stratum I and II Abilities

Subtest	Stratum I	Stratum II
Symbolic Memory	MV	Gv
Spatial Memory	MV, SR	Gv
Object Memory	MV	Gv
Cube Design	RG	Gf
Analogic Reasoning	I	Gf
Mazes	SS	Gv

Note. Gv = Visual Processing; Gf = Fluid Intelligence; MV = Visual Memory; SR = Spatial Relations; RG = Quantitative Reasoning; I = Induction; and SS = Spatial Scanning.

Goals for UNIT Development

According to Bracken and McCallum (1998), ten goals guided the development of the UNIT. The overarching goal was to ensure a fair assessment of intelligence for those children and adolescents whose cognitive and intellectual abilities cannot be adequately or fairly assessed with language-loaded measures or with existing unidimensional nonverbal measures. These individuals include those who are Deaf or hard of hearing, those from different cultural backgrounds, those who have learning/language disabilities, those with speech impairments, and those with serious emotional or intellectual limitations. The UNIT was designed to be administered in a (100%) nonverbal format, and was standardized accordingly, the only multidimensional nonverbal test so developed. See Rapid Reference 3.2 for a brief list of the 10 UNIT development goals.

Description of the UNIT

Several scores can be calculated for the UNIT total test, including a Full Scale score (FSIQ), Memory Quotient (MQ), Reasoning Quotient (RQ), Symbolic Quotient

---

⟰ Rapid Reference 3.2

Ten UNIT Development Goals

1. Ensure fairness by minimizing/eliminating known sources of bias
2. Assess intelligence with psychometric rigor and precision
3. Incorporate tasks that maximize existing examiner knowledge and experience
4. Encourage efficient administration by including three assessment options
5. Include examinee-friendly tasks
6. Assess important cognitive subdomains: memory and reasoning, symbolic and nonsymbolic organization
7. Assess psychometric g well
8. Use a 100% nonverbal administration format
9. Use a 100% nonverbal response format
10. Create a socially sensitive measure for cross-cultural assessment

(SQ), and Nonsymbolic Quotient (NSQ). Individual subtest scores can be derived for each of the six subtests for further analysis of an examinee's performance. UNIT subtests are described below. The first three subtests are designed to assess memory; the last three are designed to assess reasoning. The subtests are:

- Symbolic Memory: the examinee recalls and recreates sequences of visually presented universal symbols (e.g., green boy, black woman).
- Spatial Memory: the examinee must remember and recreate the placement of black and/or green chips on a 3 × 3 or 4 × 4 cell grid.
- Object Memory: the examinee is shown a visual array of common objects (e.g., shoe, telephone, tree) for five seconds, after which the examinee identifies the pictured objects from a larger array of pictured objects.
- Cube Design: the examinee completes three-dimensional block designs using between one and nine green and white blocks.
- Analogic Reasoning: the examinee completes matrix analogies employing common objects (e.g., hand/glove, foot/_____?) and novel geometric figures.
- Mazes: the examinee completes mazes by tracing a path through each maze from the center starting point to an exit.

DON'T FORGET

Scores available from the UNIT

Global Scores	Subtest Scores
Full Scale IQ (FSIQ)	Symbolic Memory
Memory Quotient (MQ)	Cube Design
Reasoning Quotient (RQ)	Spatial Memory
Symbolic Quotient (SQ)	Analogic Reasoning
Nonsymbolic Quotient (NSQ)	Object Memory
	Mazes

Note. Global scores use a mean set to 100 and a standard deviation set to 15; subtest scores use a mean set to 10 and a standard deviation set to 3.

Standardization and Psychometric Properties of the UNIT

Standardization of the UNIT was based on data from 2,100 children from ages 5 years 0 months through 17 years 11 months 30 days; the sample was chosen based on a carefully designed, stratified, random selection. Consequently, the data were closely representative of the U.S. population. Stratification variables included sex, race, Hispanic origin, region, community setting, classroom placement, special education status, and parental educational attainment. There were 175 children in each of 12 age groups. An additional 1,765 children and adolescents participated in related reliability, validity, and fairness studies.

The average internal consistency reliability estimates were computed for subtests and global scores for the standardization sample *and* for a combined clinical/exceptional sample. The median of the average subtest reliability coefficients across ages is .83 for the Standard Battery and .80 for the Extended Battery, with average subtest reliability coefficients across age groups ranging from .64 (Mazes) to .91 (Cube Design). Coefficients for the clinical/exceptional sample are uniformly higher, ranging from .82 (Mazes) to .96 (Cube Design). The average reliability coefficients for the global scores from the Standard Battery range from .87 (Symbolic) to .91 (Nonsymbolic) for the standardization sample; from the Extended Battery the coefficients range from .86 (Reasoning) to .90 (Memory) for the standardization sample. Coefficients for the Full Scale IQ ranged from .91 to .98 across all Batteries and the two samples. Importantly, full scale reliability coefficients need to be above .90 if they are to be used for making selection/placement decisions (see Bracken, 1987; Bracken & McCallum, 1998).

To help ensure fairness, internal consistency estimates are reported in the *UNIT Manual* for special populations (e.g., children with learning disabilities or speech and language impairments) and for important decision-making points (i.e., FSIQ of 70 plus or minus 10, and 130 plus or minus 10). Obtained coefficients and those corrected for restriction and expansion in range are reported. In general, these coefficients are impressive, and are comparable to those reported for the standardization sample. Average coefficients across ages are reported in Rapid Reference 3.3 for subtests and global scores for the two samples.

Test-retest stability was assessed using a sample of 197 participants who took the UNIT twice over an interval of approximately three weeks. Average test-retest practice effects are gains of 7.2 points for the Abbreviated Battery, 5.0 points for the Standard Battery, and 4.8 points for the Extended Battery.

≡Rapid Reference 3.3

Average Internal Consistency Reliability Coefficients for Subtests and Global Scores

UNIT Subtest or Scale	Standardization Sample	Clinical/Exceptional Sample
Abbreviated Battery FSIQ	.91	.96
Standard Battery FSIQ	.93	.98
Extended Battery FSIQ	.93	.98
Standard Battery Memory	.88	.95
Standard Battery Reasoning	.90	.96
Standard Battery Symbolic	.87	.95
Standard Battery Nonsymbolic	.91	.97
Extended Battery Memory	.90	.96
Extended Battery Reasoning	.86	.95
Extended Battery Symbolic	.89	.96
Extended Battery Nonsymbolic	.87	.95
Symbolic Memory	.85	.92
Cube Design	.91	.96
Spatial Memory	.81	.92
Analogic Reasoning	.79	.91
Object Memory	.76	.91
Mazes	.64	.82

Obtained coefficients and those corrected for restriction and expansion in range are reported in the *Manual.* Corrected subtest coefficients range from .58 (Mazes) to .85 (Cube Design), and corrected global coefficients range from .78 to .88. Coefficients for Full Scale IQs across the three batteries range from .83 (Abbreviated Battery) to .88 (Standard Battery).

The *UNIT Manual* presents results from several validity studies. Construct validity is examined using both exploratory and confirmatory factor analytic results, as well as model-testing statistics. Factor loadings from these analyses yield support for the theoretical and conceptual model of the UNIT. For example, g loadings from five of the six subtests are above .70, the value Kaufman and Lichtenberger (1999) describe as "good." Loadings of this magnitude provide good evidence for the ability of the UNIT to assess g, one of the 10 developmental goals. Additional factor analytic results provide support for the Reasoning and Memory factors, as well as the symbolic and nonsymbolic components (Bracken & McCallum, 1998).

Correlational studies with other measures of intelligence provide external evidence of construct validity. For example, coefficients showing the relationship between the Wechsler Intelligence Scale–Third Edition (WISC-III; Wechsler, 1991) and the UNIT Standard Battery FSIQs across four populations (e.g., children with learning disabilities, mental retardation) ranged from .81 to .84. The corrected correlations between the UNIT FSIQs and the Woodcock Johnson–Revised (Woodcock & Johnson, 1989) Broad Cognitive Ability score are .80, .83, and .82, respectively, for the Abbreviated, Standard, and Extended batteries for a sample of 88 examinees in regular education classes. The correlation between the Kaufman Brief Intelligence Test (K-BIT; Kaufman & Kaufman, 1990) FSIQ and the UNIT Abbreviated Battery, both screening tests, is .71 for a sample of 31 examinees. Coefficients between the UNIT Standard Battery FSIQ and three matrices-based tests are .50 (Raven's SPM; Raven, 1960), .68 (TONI-II; Brown, Sherbenou, & Johnsen, 1990) and .79 (MAT Total Test Standard Score; Naglieri, 1985). Additional validity studies are reported in the *Manual* showing relationships between the UNIT and various achievement test scores across several populations; most of these coefficients range from .25 to .50, with a few exceptions below and above this range.

One of the unique features of the UNIT is the inclusion of an entire chapter in the Examiner's Manual focusing on fairness. This chapter describes early development efforts to reduce bias, such as the use of expert bias panels to eliminate faulty items. In addition, the chapter shows reliability and internal and external validity data for several populations of interest to UNIT examiners (e.g., African Americans, Hispanic Americans, Native Americans, Asian Americans, Ecuadorians, and individuals with hearing impairments). For example, reliability coefficients for all global scale scores are in the .90s across four different populations. Of interest to many users of nonverbal tests are mean difference analyses showing average FSIQ differences between minority populations and matched nonminority samples. For example, the Standard Battery FSIQ average for a sample of 352

African Americans is 90.68; Table 6.4 in the *UNIT Manual* compares that score to the mean obtained from a matched sample of white examinees drawn from the standardization sample (99.31), a difference of 8.63. The difference between a sample of Hispanic examinees and matched controls is 2.13, which is less than the UNIT Standard Error of Measurement. See Rapid Reference 3.4 for the mean differences obtained in samples from eight populations.

Considerable effort was expended to establish fairness for the populations of interest to users of nonverbal tests. McCallum (1999) describes 13 criteria the UNIT authors used to establish fairness for the test. This effort is unmatched by any other available nonverbal test and represents a decided strength for the UNIT.

HOW TO ADMINISTER AND SCORE THE UNIT

According to the *UNIT Manual*, examiners will likely be psychologists (e.g., clinical, school, or neuropsychologists), certified specialists (educational diag-

≡Rapid Reference 3.4

UNIT Standard Battery FSIQ Mean Difference Comparisons across Eight Populations

Mean Difference Score	Effect Size	Matched Comparison Group
0.49	.03	Male Examinees/Female Examinees
8.63	.58	African-Americans/Whites
9.41*	.63	Asian Americans or Pacific Islanders/Whites
6.50	.43	Native Americans/Whites
2.13	.14	Hispanics/Non-Hispanics
3.56	.24	Bilingual or ESL Individuals/White Non-Hispanics
6.20	.41	Deaf Individuals/Individuals without hearing loss
5.33	.36	Ecuadorian examinees/U.S. examinees

*The direction of the difference favors the minority group.

nosticians, psychometrists), or those in other fields who are certified to use measures of intelligence. Users are encouraged to practice within their scope of expertise and to adhere to the ethical guidelines supplied by professional organizations such as the American Psychological Association and reported in documents such as the *Standards for Educational and Psychological Testing* (1999). Graduate training in measurement, psychological assessment, and foundations of psychology is typically considered necessary. Additional specific guidelines are suggested, including reading the *Manual*, viewing a training video available from the publisher, administering a practice case, and so forth.

Successful administration of the UNIT requires that the examiner consider three elements: the examinee, the examiner, and the physical and psychological environment. The *UNIT Manual* describes in detail considerations associated with all three elements (Bracken & McCallum, 1998).

Because the UNIT was developed to be sensitive to *examinees* from different cultures and with various disabilities, the *UNIT Manual* devotes several pages to the unique needs associated with these populations (e.g., individuals from different cultures, individuals with limited English proficiency, and individuals with speech and language impairments). For example, examiners must learn as much as possible about the characteristics, mores, and beliefs of culturally different examinees. In some cultures little value is placed on speeded responses, with more emphasis placed on pensive, reflective strategies. In addition, some individuals with physical disabilities may be able to respond to the task demands of some UNIT subtests, but not others (e.g., the Cube Design subtest requires motoric manipulation, but the Analogic Reasoning subtest requires only pointing). Examiners must be aware of the examinees' characteristics and the extent to which these characteristics mesh with task demands of the UNIT.

The *examiner*'s characteristics are also very important. A well-trained and sensitive examiner is essential for a valid assessment. Examiners must be able to establish rapport, follow standardization directions carefully, be aware of the unique administration demands of the UNIT (e.g., administration gestures, use of pantomime, time constraints), and be aware of the physical demands (e.g., positioning of the examiner/examinee depending on the handedness of the examinee). The *UNIT Manual* provides graphics to guide the placement of test materials and the examinee/examiner relative to those materials. Of course, good examiners are aware of the need to use the language of the child or employing gestures to maintain motivation (e.g., gesturing "thumbs up" for effort, saying "good job"). Importantly, examiners have considerable latitude in communicating the nature of the task demands to the examinee, through the use of gestures and pantomime, and through demonstration, sample, and checkpoint items. Each subtest uses a simple point-wave-shrug sequence. That is, the examiner points to the stimulus materials, uses the hand wave to highlight the response materials, and uses the open-handed shrug to communicate to the examinee the need to respond.

Environmental characteristics are also important. As mentioned above, the examiner should be aware of the particular needs/requirements of certain subtests, such as the use of a stopwatch, placement on the tables of certain blocks during particular items of the Cube Design subtest, and so forth. Of course, general awareness of environmental needs is also important and includes considerations such as use of a table matched to the size of the child; the need for a quiet, well-lit room; or the placement of a third person into the environment (i.e., a foreign-language or American Sign Language interpreter). Facilitation of a good psychological environment is also important. Examinees should be comfortable, yet motivated. Rapid Reference 3.5 summarizes the needed examiner, examinee, and environmental characteristics.

Starting and Discontinuing Subtests

Each subtest has two starting points, one for 5-year 0-month to 7-year 11-month-old children, and a second for examinees eight and older. Starting points for each subtest are clearly indicated on the UNIT Record Booklet, as are the discontinue rules. Specific discontinue rules are indicated in Rapid References 3.6 to 3.11.

Test Booklets

The UNIT Test Booklet provides correct responses for all subtests, as well as indications of starting points, designation of item type (i.e., demonstration, sample, checkpoint, or regular), and time limits for the two subtests for which time is critical. Also in the Test Booklet are worksheets allowing the examiner to convert raw scores to standard scores easily. The back page of the UNIT Record Booklet contains the Interpretive Worksheet, which provides a number of graphics in "tabular form" to allow testing of various hypotheses. Many

≡*Rapid Reference 3.5*

Summary of Examiner, Examinee, and Environmental Needs

Examinee Needs

Appropriate test session (e.g., well-lit room, appropriately sized furniture)
Necessary motivation (e.g., well fed, adequate sleep)
Means of communicating with examiner

Examiner Needs

Training in nonverbal administration according to UNIT *Manual* (e.g., familiarity with gestures, use of teaching items)
Familiarity with scoring criteria, time constraints, subtest demands
Familiarity with physical needs of examinee and with room characteristics
Familiarity with unique language and cultural needs of examinee
Capacity to establish and maintain rapport

Environmental Needs

Appropriate match between size of examinee and room furniture
Appropriate lighting, temperature, noise level
Appropriate rapport to facilitate psychological environment

comparisons are possible, including comparisons among global scale scores, comparisons of subtest scores to the mean of all subtests, comparisons of subtest scores to means obtained from specific scales, and comparisons of pairs of subtests. Comparisons can be made at different levels of statistical confidence by referring to the *UNIT Manual,* and the level of confidence chosen may be entered on the Interpretive Worksheet.

All subtests are dichotomously scored, with two exceptions—Cube Design and Mazes. With the exception of the first two items, each item from the Cube Design subtest is scored 1, 2, or 3 depending on the correct placement of the block designs along three axes (i.e., using a three-dimensional scoring system, one point may be earned for each axis or facet). The Mazes subtest, included on a separate booklet, is also scored uniquely, based on the number of correct decision points traversed by the examinee before the examinee's first error.

Each correct decision point is awarded one point credit, and correct decision points are shown on the Test Booklet.

Timing

Because many cultures do not place great value on speeded performance, speed is deemphasized on the UNIT. Only two of the subtests, Cube Design and Mazes, provide bonus points for speed; even then, bonus points for speed never exceed two points for any Cube Design item and three points for any Mazes item. Bonus points are clearly indicated on the Test Booklet. Time of response is not critical on any other subtest, although all three memory subtests require that presentation of the stimulus materials be limited to five seconds. It is recommended that examiners start their stopwatches and let them run during presentation of the stimulus items on the three memory subtests: Symbolic Memory, Spatial Memory, and Object Memory. There is no need for a stopwatch for the Analogic Reasoning subtest.

Item Types

There are four items types. Demonstration items are presented by the examiner and are not scored. Sample items are completed by the examinee, with feedback from the examiner if needed; they too are not scored. Checkpoint items are completed by the examinee and scored; feedback is provided if the item is failed. Regular items are completed by the examinee and scored; no feedback is allowed. Each item type is clearly identified in the UNIT Test Booklet.

Subtest-by-Subtest Rules of Administration

UNIT norms allow for administration of a two-, four-, or six-subtest battery. Completion of the six-subtest Extended Battery requires approximately 45 minutes. The two-subtest Abbreviated Battery takes about 15 minutes to administer; the four-subtest Standard Battery requires about 30 minutes. The Standard Battery is recommended for most purposes, including assessment leading to placement decisions.

Like other standardized tests, administration of the UNIT produces norm-referenced scores that represent an individual's performance relative to the performance of same-age peers. In order to obtain test results that can be compared with confidence to the data collected during standardization, and by inference to all same-age peers in the United States, it is necessary to carefully adhere to the same test administration procedures used during standardization. Unlike most other intelligence tests, all items from the UNIT must be administered completely nonverbally—using gestures, pantomime, and modeling—as described in the *UNIT Manual*. Consequently, learning to administer the test requires mastery of some unique nonverbal skills. Only those examiners who have had proper training and experience should administer the test. Those individuals who have had formal graduate-level coursework in the administration and interpretation of individualized standardized cognitive tests may use the UNIT. With training in standardized testing, these individuals can acquire the necessary administration skills by reading the *Manual,* viewing a training video, and practicing administration. Because administration must be nonverbal, there are detailed verbal directions and ample graphics in the *Manual;* in addition, there are supplemental training materials available including the training video mentioned above, a Training Guide for individual and classroom use (Bracken & McCallum, 1999), and a training CD. In addition, each kit comes with an $8\frac{1}{2} \times 11$-inch laminated sheet called "Administration at a Glance"; on this sheet are brief subtest directions and pictures of the gestures. This guide provides the examiner with a brief reminder of the administration requirements for each subtest.

Even though UNIT administration is somewhat unique, it is not difficult. The examiner models completion of the demonstration items and provides feedback on the sample items when necessary. A unique feature of the UNIT is the inclusion of checkpoint items; these items provide an additional opportunity for the examiner to provide feedback. In addition, the eight gestures used during administration are very common and are easy for examinees to understand (e.g., nodding or "thumbs up" for yes or good effort, head shaking for no). The typical administration strategy for all subtests begins with the examiner ensuring that the examinee makes eye contact, presenting the stimulus materials, pointing to the materials, waving his/her hand over the response options and materials, and shrugging (using the open-handed shrugging gesture). See Figure 3.1 for a display of the gestures.

Though UNIT administration is nonverbal, it should not be stilted or artificial. Examiners can and should talk to examinees to establish and maintain

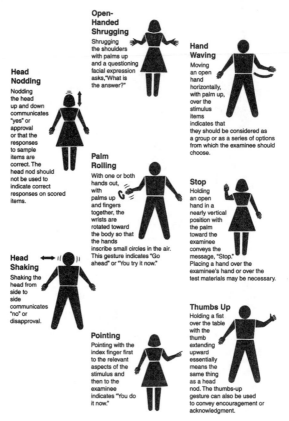

Head Nodding

Nodding the head up and down communicates "yes" or approval or that the responses to sample items are correct. The head nod should not be used to indicate correct responses on scored items.

Head Shaking

Shaking the head from side to side communicates "no" or disapproval.

Open-Handed Shrugging

Shrugging the shoulders with palms up and a questioning facial expression asks,"What is the answer?"

Palm Rolling

With one or both hands out, with palms up and fingers together, the wrists are rotated toward the body so that the hands inscribe small circles in the air. This gesture indicates "Go ahead" or "You try it now."

Pointing

Pointing with the index finger first to the relevant aspects of the stimulus and then to the examinee indicates "You do it now."

Hand Waving

Moving an open hand horizontally, with palm up, over the stimulus items indicates that they should be considered as a group or as a series of options from which the examinee should choose.

Stop

Holding an open hand in a nearly vertical position with the palm toward the examinee conveys the message, "Stop." Placing a hand over the examinee's hand or over the test materials may be necessary.

Thumbs Up

Holding a fist over the table with the thumb extending upward essentially means the same thing as a head nod. The thumbs-up gesture can also be used to convey encouragement or acknowledgment.

Figure 3.1 UNIT Administration Gestures

rapport if there is a common language. It is helpful to talk to examinees to establish rapport, to obtain background information, and so on. However, the examiner *may not* talk to the examinee about UNIT test directions or responses.

Each UNIT subtest requires that the examiner present the stimulus material nonverbally. For the *Symbolic Memory* subtest, stimulus plates are presented on an easel. The easel contains plates showing pictures of one or more of the following universal human figures, in a particular order (e.g., a green baby, a black baby, a green girl, a black girl, a green boy, a black boy, a green woman, a black woman, a green man, and a black man). The examinee is presented the stimulus plate for five seconds, then is instructed through modeling and gestures to replicate the

≡Rapid Reference 3.6

Summary of Symbolic Memory Rules

Starting Points

Examinees aged 5 to 7 begin with Demonstration 1.

Examinees aged 8 to 17 begin with Demonstration 4.

Timing

Each item is presented for 5 seconds; responses are not timed.

Discontinue Criterion

Discontinue after scores of 0 on both items 1 and 2 or after five consecutive scores of 0 on items 2–30.

Reversal Rules

If an examinee aged 8 to 17 receives a score of 0 on Sample 4, testing resumes with Demonstration 1.

order shown on the stimulus plate. The examinee uses $1\frac{1}{2}'' \times 1\frac{1}{2}''$ response cards, each containing one of the universal human figures, to reproduce the array depicted on the stimulus plate. The task has no time limits and no bonus credit for rapid performance. Materials needed include Stimulus Book 1, 10 Symbolic Memory Response Cards, and a stopwatch. Rapid Reference 3.6 reviews the starting, reversal, and discontinue rules and the guidelines for timing.

The *Cube Design* subtest requires the examinee to use up to nine cubes to replicate two- or three-dimensional designs shown on a stimulus plate. A Response Mat provides a work space for constructing the designs, and presents a diagonal line to allow the examinee to orient placement. Each cube contains six facets: two white sides, two green sides, and two sides that contain diagonals (triangles), one green and one white. These cubes can be arranged to replicate the two- and three-dimensional figures depicted on the stimulus plates. Items 1 and 2 are scored on two-dimension (facet) only; items 3 through 15 are scored on each facet of three-dimensional figures. Items are timed but the time limits are liberal to emphasize the power, rather than speeded nature, of the task. Materials needed for the subtest include Stimulus Book 1, nine green and white Cube Design cubes, Cube Design Response Mat, and a stopwatch. Examiners should remember that for items 1 and 2, the response cube is presented so that the correct face for completing the design is *not* up. For item 3, the response cube is presented with a solid white face up. For items 4 and 5, one cube is presented with a solid face up and one with a two-color face up. For items 6–15, the cubes are scrambled and presented so that at least one of each face is up. For each item the examiner presents the correct number of cubes needed to complete the design. This number is presented in parentheses on the Test Booklet. Rapid Reference 3.7 outlines the starting, stopping, and reversal rules and the timing guidelines.

For the *Spatial Memory* subtest the examiner presents a stimulus plate showing a random pattern of green and black dots on a 3 × 3 or 4 × 4 grid. After viewing the stimulus for 5 seconds, the examinee recreates the pattern by placing green and black circular chips on a response grid. The examiner does not allow the examinee to touch the chips until the stimulus plate has been covered. Materials needed for this subtest includes Stimulus Book 1, 16 Response Chips (8 green, 8 black), Response Grid (3 × 3 on one side and 4 × 4 on the

═Rapid Reference 3.7

Summary of Cube Design Rules

Starting Points

Examinees aged 5 to 7 begin with Demonstration 1.

Examinees aged 8 to 17 begin with the response mat page immediately preceding Demonstration 3.

Timing

Examinees have 60 seconds to complete each for items 1–5 and 120 seconds for each item for items 6–15.

Discontinue Criterion

Discontinue after scores of 0 on both items 1 and 2 or after three consecutive scores of 0 on items 2–15.

Reversal Rules

If an examinee aged 8 to 17 receives a score of 0 on Sample 3, testing resumes with Demonstration 1.

Rapid Reference 3.8

Summary of Spatial Memory Rules

Starting Points

Examinees aged 5 to 7 begin with Demonstration 1.

Examinees aged 8 to 17 begin with Demonstration 5.

Timing

Each item is presented for 5 seconds; responses are not timed.

Discontinue Criteria

Discontinue after scores of 0 on both items for 1 and 2 or after five consecutive scores of 0 on items 2–27.

Reversal Rules

If an examinee aged 8 to 17 receives a score of 0 on Sample 5, testing resumes with Demonstration 1.

other), and a stopwatch. See Rapid Reference 3.8 for the starting, reversal, and stopping rules and for timing guidelines.

The Analogic Reasoning subtest requires the examinee to solve analogies presented in a matrix format. The examinee is directed to indicate which one of several options best completes a two-cell or a four-cell analogy. Task solution requires the examinee to determine the relationships between objects. For example, in the four-cell matrix, the first cell might depict a fish and the second water; the third cell might show a bird, and the fourth cell would be blank. The examinee would select from several options the picture that best completes the matrix. In this case a picture of the sky would be a correct response. Materials needed for this subtest include Stimulus Book 1. See Rapid Reference 3.9 for the starting, reversal, and stopping rules and the timing guidelines.

For the *Object Memory* subtest, the examiner presents pictures of common objects arranged on stimulus plates located on an administration easel. The easel is laid flat on the table and the examinee is shown a plate containing pictures of one or more objects for five seconds. The examinee is then shown a second plate containing pictures from the first plate and pictures of "distractor objects." The examinee identifies pictures on the second plate that were

≣*Rapid Reference 3.9*

Summary of Analogic Reasoning Rules

Starting Points
Examinees aged 5 to 7 begin with Demonstration 1.
Examinees aged 8 to 17 begin with Demonstration 4.

Timing
This subtest is not timed.

Discontinue Criterion
Discontinue after scores of 0 on both items for 1 and 2 or after four scores of 0 in five consecutive items on items 2–31.

Reversal Rules
If an examinee aged 8 to 17 receives a score of 0 on Sample 4, testing resumes with Demonstration 1.

shown on the first plate; to create a semipermanent response, the examinee places black chips on the pictures selected. The examiner should not allow the examinee to touch the response chips until after the stimulus page has been turned. This memory task is not timed, other than the 5-second stimulus exposure. Materials needed for this subtest include Stimulus Book 2, eight black Response Chips, and a stopwatch. See Rapid Reference 3.10 for the starting, reversal, and stopping rules and the timing guidelines.

The *Mazes* subtest requires the examinee to complete a maze using a number two lead pencil, minus the eraser. The examinee demonstrates successful completion initially, using a red-leaded pencil. Each maze shows a mouse in the center and one or more pieces of cheese on the outside of the maze. The cheese depicts one or more possible exits from the maze. The task is to determine the correct path from the center to the (correct) piece of cheese. The examinee is stopped immediately after making the first error, and the examinee is given one point credit for each correct decision up to the point of the first error. The Test Booklet shows successfully completed mazes and indicates correct decision points. Errors include entering a blind alley, crossing a wall, and retracing. Neither passing through a wall while rounding a corner nor briefly crossing a wall and returning to the alley is counted as an error. Exam-

≡ *Rapid Reference 3.10*

Summary of Object Memory Rules

Starting Points

Examinees aged 5 to 7 begin with Demonstration 1.

Examinees aged 8 to 17 begin with Demonstration 2.

Timing

Each item is presented for 5 seconds; responses are not timed.

Discontinue Criterion

Discontinue after scores of 0 on both items 1 and 2 or after five consecutive scores of 0 on items 2–30.

Reversal Rules

If an examinee aged 8 to 17 receives a score of 0 on Sample 2, testing resumes with Demonstration 1.

iners are instructed to give the examinee the benefit of the doubt in borderline cases. Items are timed, though the time limits are quite liberal, and one to three bonus points are possible for rapid performance on items 9 through 13. If the examinee stops before completing any maze the examiner uses gestures to encourage completion. Materials needed for this subtest include the Mazes Response Booklet, a number 2 graphite pencil without eraser, a red-leaded pencil, and a stopwatch. See Rapid Reference 3.11 for the starting, reversal, and stopping rules and for timing guidelines.

UNIT INTERPRETATION

The UNIT allows three administration options: the Abbreviated two-subtest battery, the Standard four-subtest battery, and the Extended six-subtest battery. All UNIT batteries were designed to assess memory and reasoning as well as symbolic and nonsymbolic processing.

Interpretation begins with the examiner's consideration of which battery should be administered. Making a choice among the three batteries depends on several issues, including the purpose of the assessment (e.g., screening, di-

≡ Rapid Reference 3.11

Summary of Mazes Rules

Starting Points

Examinees aged 5 to 7 begin with Demonstration 1.
Examinees aged 8 to 17 begin with Demonstration 3.

Timing

Examinees have 60 seconds to complete items 1–8, and 120 seconds for items 9–13. Bonus points are possible for items 9–13.

Discontinue Criterion

Discontinue after a combined raw score of 0 or 1 on three consecutive scored mazes.

Reversal Rules

If an examinee aged 8 to 17 receives less than full credit on Sample 3, testing resumes with Demonstration 1.

---

agnostic testing, placement), the estimated attention span of the student, the time available to conduct the assessment, and related concerns. Once the choice of batteries has been made and the UNIT has been administered, actual test interpretation is conducted in multiple steps that consider data successively from the most global and reliable sources (e.g., FSIQ, scale scores) to increasingly more specific, yet less reliable sources (e.g., subtests, items).

The current literature on intelligence test interpretation focuses primarily on two types of interpretive strategies, normative and ipsative. Kaufman (1979, 1994) described a logical and systematic approach for interpreting the Wechsler scales from both an interchild (normative) and intrachild (ipsative) process. Both procedures have been employed by a variety of authors (Bracken, 1984, 1998a; Kaufman & Kaufman, 1983; Elliott, 1986; McCallum, 1991; McGrew, 1996; Sattler, 1988) and have become common practice among clinical and school psychologists. Recently, McDermott and Glutting (1997) have questioned the utility of ipsative subtest analysis and have argued for the use of another interpretive strategy linked to the base rates of subtest profiles found among individuals in a test's normative sample. The following discussion for in-

DON'T FORGET

Three Administration Options

Abbreviated Battery	Standard Battery	Extended Battery
Symbolic Memory	Symbolic Memory	Symbolic Memory
Cube Design	Cube Design	Cube Design
	Spatial Memory	Spatial Memory
	Analogic Reasoning	Analogic Reasoning
		Object Memory
		Mazes

Note. The Abbreviated Battery is best suited for screening, the Standard Battery for placement decisions, and the Extended Battery for placement *and* diagnostic purposes.

terpreting the UNIT focuses primarily on the use of normative and ipsative strategies, and is adapted from guidelines recommended by Kaufman for interpreting the Wechsler Adult Intelligence Scale–Third Edition (Kaufman & Lichtenberger, 1999); these guidelines are similar to the guidelines outlined in the *UNIT Manual* (Bracken & McCallum, 1998). The strategies we suggest do include some attention to determining base rates of very common profiles in a manner similar to that recommended by McDermott and Glutting, but our suggested procedures are not as inclusive. In our clinical experience, we have found the normative and ipsative strategies we recommend to be most helpful for examining an individual's cognitive strengths and weaknesses.

General Interpretation Guidelines

Traditional normative and ipsative interpretation should proceed from the most global and reliable scores to the most specific, least reliable scores. Test composites (e.g., FSIQs and scale scores) tend to be the most reliable scores because they include sources of variation from all of the subtests and scales that comprise the test. As such, these molar data sources are more reliable than the more molecular scores that result from individual subtests. Composite cognitive ability scores also are the best predictors of important real world outcomes, particularly academic and vocational success (Sattler, 1992). Conse-

DON'T FORGET

Six Steps of UNIT Interpretation

1. Interpret the Full Scale IQ
2. Determine the statistical significance of global score differences
3. Determine whether the differences between global scores are abnormally large
4. Interpret the significant strengths and weakness of the profile
5. Interpret subtest abilities
6. Generate hypotheses about fluctuation in the UNIT profile

quently, the most defensible interpretive strategy might be to address the overall composite score and stop the interpretive process.

However, whenever there is considerable variability in an examinee's performance across individual subtests in a battery, the overall composite may not yield a good reflection of an examinee's true *overall* ability. When significant subtest and scale variation occurs, further interpretation of the test is warranted (Kaufman, 1979, 1999). Therefore, the UNIT interpretation scheme presented below follows the logical sequence of interpreting the instrument from the Full Scale IQ, the Scales, and finally the subtests.

The Six Steps of UNIT Interpretation

Step 1: Interpret the Full Scale IQ   The first stage of UNIT interpretation requires describing the examinee's performance at the composite level (i.e., Full Scale) in both quantitative (e.g., standard scores, confidence intervals, percentile ranks) and qualitative (e.g., intelligence classifications) fashion. Quantitative descriptions are based on interpretation of obtained scores relative to population parameters. For example, the UNIT composite standard scores are based on a population mean of 100 and a standard deviation of 15. As such, approximately 68% of examinees in the normative sample obtained Full Scale scores between 85 and 115; approximately 95% achieved scores between 70 and 130; and slightly more than 99% of the sample attained scores between 55 and 145. Because intelligence is a construct that conforms fairly closely to the traditional normal bell curve, standard scores on the UNIT scales can be compared to IQs and other standardized scores obtained on other tests based on the same metric (i.e., M = 100, SD = 15), such as the various Wechsler scales and the Woodcock-Johnson Psycho-Educational Battery–Revised. In addition to standard scores, the *UNIT Manual* provides percentile ranks for all scale and subtest scores.

Variability in obtained scores comes from two sources, reliable variance and error variance, and the error associated with the composite scores should be considered and communicated to clarify the difference between the examinee's obtained scores and his or her "hypothetical true scores." Because error is assumed to be normally distributed, obtained scores should be considered within a band of confidence that frames the obtained score by one or more standard error(s) of measurement (SEm), as determined by the level of confidence desired (e.g., 68%, 95%, 99%). Confidence intervals built around obtained scores define the probability that a given range of scores would include the examinee's "true" score. A true score is defined as the hypothetical average that would be obtained upon repeated testing, minus the effects of error, such as practice or fatigue. In addition to the SEm, the UNIT also reports the band of error associated with the "estimated true score." This band of error takes into account regression to the mean, so the band becomes more elliptical as scores move toward the extremes. For the UNIT, the recommended band of error (standard error of the estimate) can be found in Table B.10 in the *Manual*. Finally, qualitative descriptions are possible using the classifications provided in the *UNIT Manual* in Table B.10 also. These classifications are broad descriptions of the child's level of intellectual functioning, ranging from Very Superior to Very Delayed.

Step 2: Determine the Statistical Significance of Global Score Differences The UNIT Full Scale IQ is the first score to be interpreted because it is typically the best representation of the examinee's overall or global intelligence. However, whenever there is significant variability in an examinee's subtest and/or scale scores, the FSIQ may not serve as a good representation of global ability. To determine the representativeness of the FSIQ as an estimate of overall intellectual ability, the examiner should first consider the comparability of the UNIT scale scores (i.e., Reasoning Quotient, Memory Quotient, Symbolic Quotient, or Nonsymbolic Quotient). If scale scores show considerable variability (i.e., significant difference among themselves), these differences should be interpreted *if* they are also abnormally large (see Step 3).

How large should differences between scale scores be before the differences are considered important? If the difference between two scales is statistically significant, that is, so large that it would not likely occur by chance alone, such a difference should be considered important, at least initially. With Kaufman and Lichtenberger (1999), we recommend that a probability level of .05 be used to determine significance; however, some examiners may choose a more conservative criterion (e.g., .01). Nevertheless, statistically significant differences are not necessarily clinically meaningful or rare. If differences exist, they should be checked to determine how rare they are in the population. See Rapid Reference 3.12 for values considered significant for the Standard and Extended Batteries by age, and Rapid Reference 3.13 to determine "rareness" as described in Step 3 below.

Step 3: Determine Whether the Differences between Global Scores are Abnormally Large
The relative frequency with which significant score differences occur within the population is another important indicator of variability. Relative frequency of differences addresses a separate issue from statistical significance. As mentioned above, statistical significance is described as the probability that the obtained score difference would be expected to occur in the population by chance alone. However, differences of that magnitude may occur in the normative population with considerable frequency due to real differences in the abilities of individuals within the population, rather than to chance factors. Also, differences occur in both directions. Examiners should check Rapid Reference 3.13 to find the relative frequency of score differences in the population for differences ranging from 5 to 25. We recommend that differences exceeding 20 points be considered "abnormally large" because they typically occur only in the most extreme 15% of the population (see Naglieri & Kaufman, 1983) . If there are one or more abnormally large differences among the scale scores (e.g., Memory Quotient is significantly higher than Reasoning Quotient, Symbolic Quotient is significantly higher than Nonsymbolic Quotient), the resulting UNIT FSIQ is a less than optimal index of the examinee's overall abilities. Consequently, scales should be interpreted as important indicators of (independent) abilities in their own right. There is one caveat, however. If there is abnormal scatter among the three subtests within a particular global scale, that scale should not be interpreted as a unique and cohesive entity. Scatter is indicated by subtracting the lowest subtest score from the highest. If this range of scores is equal to or greater than six points, the scatter is abnormally large, that is, so large that only 15% of the standardization sample earned a value this large or larger.

The *UNIT Manual* provides some reasonable hypotheses describing char-

≡ Rapid Reference 3.12

Statistical Significance of Memory-Reasoning and Symbolic-Nonsymbolic Differences

Age	Standard Battery		Extended Battery	
	Memory-Reasoning	Symbolic-Nonsymbolic	Memory-Reasoning	Symbolic-Nonsymbolic
	.05 (.01)	.05 (.01)	.05 (.01)	.05 (.01)
5	16.3 (21.4)	16.2 (21.3)	15.1 (19.9)	14.6 (19.2)
6	15.9 (20.9)	16.8 (22.1)	15.1 (19.8)	15.5 (20.3)
7	16.6 (21.8)	16.4 (21.6)	15.5 (20.4)	15.8 (20.7)
8	13.0 (17.1)	13.2 (17.4)	14.8 (19.4)	14.6 (19.2)
9	14.3 (18.8)	14.9 (19.6)	15.9 (20.9)	16.0 (21.0)
10	12.7 (16.7)	13.0 (17.1)	13.6 (17.9)	13.7 (18.0)
11	13.5 (17.8)	13.9 (18.2)	14.7 (19.3)	14.9 (19.6)
12	12.6 (16.6)	12.4 (16.4)	13.7 (18.0)	13.7 (18.0)
13	12.4 (16.4)	12.3 (16.1)	13.8 (18.1)	13.6 (17.9)
14	13.3 (17.5)	13.2 (17.4)	13.9 (18.3)	13.8 (18.2)
15	13.7 (18.0)	13.9 (18.3)	14.2 (18.6)	14.3 (18.7)
16	12.5 (16.4)	12.9 (17.0)	13.2 (17.4)	13.3 (17.5)
17	13.8 (18.2)	14.0 (18.4)	14.4 (18.9)	14.4 (18.9)

Note. From Bracken and McCallum, 1998.

acteristics of examinees who have particular strengths on the global scale scores. For example, those who have greater memory than reasoning skills should be able to comprehend and reproduce visual stimuli better than they are able to problem solve based on perceived juxtapositions and relationships. Tables 3.2 through 3.5 show some of these hypotheses.

Individuals with this scale pattern may learn best through exposure to con-

Cumulative Percentages of Memory-Reasoning and Symbolic-Nonsymbolic Differences across Ages

	Standard Battery		Extended Battery	
Difference	Memory-Reasoning	Symbolic-Nonsymbolic	Memory-Reasoning	Symbolic-Nonsymbolic
25	7.4%	6.2%	6.6%	6.9%
24	9.1	8.5	8.1	8.3
23	10.9	9.5	9.6	9.2
22	11.0	9.8	10.8	10.5
21	13.3	13.1	12.4	12.3
20	16.3	14.8	15.1	14.9
19	16.4	15.4	16.9	16.2
18	19.7	19.5	20.0	19.5
17	23.2	21.8	22.7	21.3
16	23.3	23.0	25.1	23.9
15	30.4	27.4	27.9	25.8
14	34.1	29.8	32.0	29.6
13	34.4	31.7	36.0	33.3
12	41.9	36.5	40.2	37.2
11	45.8	40.3	44.5	42.4
10	46.4	43.3	48.6	45.3
9	57.6	50.6	53.9	51.3
8	60.7	55.2	57.3	54.8
7	62.0	58.6	63.0	61.2
6	72.3	66.1	67.2	66.2
5	75.4	71.6	72.9	73.0

Note. From Bracken and McCallum, 1998.

Table 3.2 Interpretive Hypotheses for Memory > Reasoning

Examinee's short-term memory skills are better developed than nonverbal reasoning.

Examinee's ability to comprehend and reproduce visual stimuli is better developed than the ability to analyze, synthesize, or reorganize visual stimuli.

Examinee's attention to relevant details is better developed than concentrated problem solving abilities.

Table 3.3 Interpretative Hypotheses for Reasoning > Memory

Examinee's nonverbal reasoning is better developed than short-term memory.

Examinee's ability to analyze, synthesize, or reorganize visual stimuli is better developed than the ability to comprehend and reproduce visual stimuli.

Examinee's ability to concentrate during problem solving activities is better than the ability to attend to relevant visual details.

Table 3.4 Interpretative Hypotheses for Symbolic > Nonsymbolic

Examinee's symbolically-mediated problem solving (using some language) is better than nonsymbolically-mediated problem solving.

Examinee's problem solving using accumulated knowledge is better than novel problem solving.

Examinee's practical tasks are more easily handled than nonpractical tasks.

Examinee's "Verbal" skills are better than "Performance" skills.

Table 3.5 Interpretative Hypotheses for Nonsymbolic > Symbolic

Examinee's nonverbal problem solving is better than symbolically-mediated problem solving (language facility).

Examinee's immediate problem solving is better than problem solving using knowledge from accumulated experience (particularly symbols of language).

Examinee may have a language deficit.

Examinee may find practical tasks more difficult than nonpractical tasks.

Examinee's "Performance" skills are better than "Verbal" skills.

crete, factual information, with memory aids, as opposed to discovery learning activities. For example, reading instruction might include considerable sight-word repetition, as opposed to a more whole language approach; instruction in higher order knowledge (e.g., comprehension, synthesis, evaluation) should be based on well-learned rules, principles, and laws (e.g., science principles, grammar rules); and learning may be aided through the use of mnemonics (e.g., "a pint's a pound the world round"). Generalizations of previously learned material to new problems or contexts might be facilitated by reminding students of basic concepts that guide problem solving (e.g., the area of complex geometric designs can be computed by reducing the design to a combination of familiar shapes, such as squares, rectangles, and triangles).

Individuals with this scale pattern may be adept at solving unique problems that are not highly dependent on previously learned information. Knowledge to be learned might best be presented through the use of relationships, comparisons, underlying principles, extrapolations, and discovery learning. Memory of information should be facilitated by assimilating new content into existing taxonomies, categories, and strategies, with an emphasis on understanding symbolic better than nonsymbolic processing.

Individuals who demonstrate better symbolic than nonsymbolic processing are more adept at using language as a means of problem solving. Through the process of subvocalization these individuals may "self-talk" their way through problem solutions. Because most academic material is symbolic in nature (e.g., reading, writing, computation), children with this scale pattern are likely to learn well in school. Information to be acquired might best be presented in a symbolic fashion (e.g., verbal, rebus, sign, gesture), such that the individual can assimilate new material into his or her own symbolic repertoire (e.g., language).

Individuals who demonstrate this scale pattern may be adept at discerning the relationships between abstract and figural stimulus characteristics. These individuals may acquire and process information especially well through nonverbal means. In new learning situations, a visual presentation (e.g., graphs, drawings) may facilitate this student's acquisition of new material. Concrete and experiential exploratory learning approaches may be especially meaningful for students with this pattern.

Step 4. Interpret the Significant Strengths and Weaknesses of the Profile   Step 4 begins the actual examination of the theoretical underpinnings of the test. That is, if the scales exhibit statistically significant and abnormally large differences, interpretation proceeds along theoretical lines (e.g., Memory greater than Reasoning, or Symbolic greater than Nonsymbolic). Examinees who also exhibit particular patterns of performance would be expected to achieve differentially, as indicated in Table 3.2. Also, non-UNIT based models may be important to consider; that possibility is investigated empirically in Step 5. For example, application of the Simultaneous-Successive model of processing, the Cattell-Horn Gf-Gc model of intelligence, or Guilford's Structure of Intellect model may shed some important light on the child's unique abilities. Using other models to explain scores should follow the same general steps outlined above. That is, the examiner might describe and define the model most suited to the test data, being careful to characterize how the pattern of scores supports the model; this step should be followed by a discussion of any subtest scores that may be incompatible with the model. Next, extra-test data should be considered to either support or refute the logic of using this particular model. Finally, the examiner is obligated to discuss how this model might be applied to explain strengths and weaknesses and the relationship between those and real world applications (e.g., educational strategies).

Step 5: Interpret Subtest Abilities   In this stage of interpretation the focus is on individual subtests. Although significant scale deviation is considered an important index, examiners should be aware that nonsignificant variability among scales does not necessarily mean that a test profile contains no significant variability. *Subtest* scores may yield statistically significant but offsetting differences that result in similar scores across scales. That is, the MQ, RQ, SQ, and NSQ may be similar, but subtests may vary significantly. Therefore, the determination of whether the FSIQ is a reasonable estimate of overall cognitive functioning is based not only on scale scores, but must be considered at the subtest level as well.

To evaluate subtest variability within scales the examiner may refer to Table D.3 in the *UNIT Manual*, in which differences required for significance between each subtest and the mean subtest scores are provided by age level. Using that Table, it is possible to compare each subtest to the mean of the scale scores, or to the entire test, at various levels of confidence. The necessary elements of Table D.3 have been excerpted in Rapid Reference 3.14.

The process of comparing individual subtest scores with the average subtest score should be completed for each scale (i.e., Memory, Reasoning, Symbolic, Nonsymbolic) and all subtests combined (i.e., all six subtests in a pooled fashion), as necessary. As previously mentioned, if scores between the global scales are not significantly or abnormally large, subtests should be compared to the overall mean in the pooled procedure, which considers the extent to

⟠Rapid Reference 3.14

Differences between Single Subtest Scores and Global Means and Differences Obtained by Various Percentages of the UNIT Standardization Sample

Scale-Subtest	Significance Level			Cumulative Percentage		
	.10	.05	.01	1%	5%	10%
	Subtest variability within scales approach (Extended Battery)					
Memory—SM	2.2	2.4	3.0	4.7	3.7	3.0
Memory—SpaM	2.3	2.6	3.2	4.7	3.3	3.0
Memory—OM	2.4	2.7	3.4	4.7	3.7	3.0
Reasoning—CD	2.1	2.3	2.8	4.7	3.7	3.0
Reasoning—AR	2.4	2.7	3.4	5.0	3.7	3.0
Reasoning—M	2.8	3.2	3.9	6.0	4.3	3.7
Symbolic—SM	2.2	2.5	3.0	5.0	3.7	3.0
Symbolic—AR	2.4	2.7	3.3	5.0	3.7	3.0
Symbolic—OM	2.5	2.8	3.4	4.7	3.7	3.0
NonSymbolic—CD	2.0	2.3	2.8	4.7	3.7	3.0
NonSymbolic—SpaM	2.4	2.6	3.2	4.7	3.7	3.0
NonSymbolic—M	2.8	3.1	3.9	5.7	4.3	3.7
Scale-Subtest	**Pooled Subtest Approach (Standard Battery)**					
Standard—SM	2.3	2.6	3.1	5.5	4.0	3.3
Standard—CD	2.0	2.2	2.7	4.8	3.8	3.0
Standard—SpaM	2.5	2.8	3.4	5.0	3.8	3.0
Standard—AR	2.6	2.9	3.5	5.5	4.0	3.3

Scale-Subtest	Significance Level			Cumulative Percentage		
	.10	.05	.01	1%	5%	10%
	Pooled Subtest Approach (Extended Battery)					
Extended—SM	2.6	2.9	3.5	5.7	4.2	3.5
Extended—CD	2.2	2.4	2.9	5.2	4.0	3.3
Extended—SpaM	2.9	3.2	3.8	5.0	3.8	3.2
Extended—AR	3.0	3.3	4.0	5.7	4.2	3.5
Extended—OM	3.2	3.5	4.2	5.5	4.3	3.5
Extended—M	3.8	4.1	4.9	6.8	5.2	4.3

Note. SM = Symbolic Memory; SpaM = Spatial Memory; OM = Object Memory; CD = Cube Design; AR = Analogic Reasoning; M = Mazes. From Bracken and McCallum, 1998

which individual subtests deviate from the overall average subtest score. The process requires that the mean of all six UNIT subtests be computed and each subtest score is individually compared to the mean of the six to identify "outliers," (i.e., scores that differ significantly from the overall subtest mean). In this case the assumption is that variability within the UNIT cannot be characterized according to the model of abilities that underpins the test (i.e., memory, reasoning, symbolic and nonsymbolic processing).

The following guidelines are required to conduct the pooled interpretive process. The examiner should: (a) average all six subtest scaled scores; (b) create deviation scores by subtracting each respective subtest score from the mean subtest score; (c) examine Rapid Reference 3.14 to identify subtests that deviate significantly from the average score (i.e., determine strengths and weaknesses); (d) examine Rapid Reference 3.15 to determine whether individual subtests possess sufficient specificity to be interpreted as measuring some unique cognitive ability; (e) consider the abilities that underpin individual subtests (Table 3.6) to begin generating hypotheses or potential explanations for individual subtest strengths and weaknesses (e.g., conflicting subtest scores, inconsistent subtest patterns); (f) reconcile strong and weak abilities by examining comparable subtests and abilities assessed by other tests administered in the battery; and (g) consider additional extra-test variables, such as the referral problem, teacher/parent reports, class and assessment behavior observations, and students' work samples to support or refute hypotheses that are generated during the interpretation process. These same guidelines can be followed for determining strengths and weaknesses within scales. For example, any subtest can be compared to its scale mean (i.e., spatial memory to the three memory subtests). The process is the same.

Step 6: Generate Hypotheses about Fluctuation in the UNIT Profile   If scores are consistent with the test model (i.e., they show little variability, or they show significant and rare memory versus reasoning or symbolic versus nonsymbolic difference), interpretation is straightforward and simple. However, such patterns are not particularly common and other models may be investigated (e.g., simultaneous versus successive, Gf, Gc). In some cases, no model-based approach will explain functioning, and individual subtest scores must be examined. Table 3.6, also found in the *UNIT Manual,* helps examiners generate hypotheses about strengths and weaknesses.

In some instances, hypotheses may be generated from the unique features of the test. Certain features of the UNIT are particularly important to consider because of the relevance of these features to interpretation. First, the UNIT is administered solely through the use of gestures and demonstration; consequently, only indirect hypotheses can be generated from test performance about the examinee's verbal skills through his or her performance on the Symbolic Scale. When writing a psychological report based on the UNIT, the examiner will have some knowledge of the student's verbal abilities from extra-test sources and these skills should be described in the background section of the report. Second, the test provides the opportunity for responses that require considerable motoric manipulation (e.g., handling blocks) as well as merely pointing to answers. Administration of the subtests can be modified so that only a pointing response is required on four of the subtests. The use of motoric and motor-reduced subtests facilitates administration by optimizing motivation and rapport. For example, a very shy child may be encouraged initially to point in response to items, and later, as more rapport is built, other, more motorically involved responses may be possible. Third, the subtests were

Table 3.6 Primary and Secondary Abilities Assessed by the Universal Nonverbal Intelligence Test

SM	CD	SpaM	AR	OM	M	Abilities
	P		P			Abstract Thinking
	P		P			Analysis
P	P	P	S	P		Attention to Detail
P	P			P	P	Concentration
S			P	S		Concept Formation
	P		P		P	Evaluation
	P					Holistic Processing
					P	Impulse Control
	P	P			P	Nonsymbolic Mediation
	P				P	Nonverbal Reasoning
					P	Paper and Pencil Manipulation
	P	P	S		S	Perception of Abstract Stimuli
P			P	P		Perception of Meaningful Stimuli
S	P	P	S	S	P	Perceptual Organization
					P	Planning Ability
	P		P		P	Reasoning
	P					Reproduction of a Model
P			S		P	Sequential Processing
	P	P	S	P		Simultaneous Processing
	P	P	S		P	Spatial Orientation
P			P	P		Symbolic Mediation
	P		P			Synthesis
	P					Three-Dimensional Representation
P			P	P		Verbal Mediation
S	P	S		S	P	Visual-Motor Integration
P			P	P		Visual Short Term Memory
	S				S	Working under Time Constraints

Note. P indicates a primary ability; S indicates a secondary ability. SM = Symbolic Memory, CD = Cube Design; SpaM = Spatial Memory; AR = Analogic Reasoning; OM = Object Memory; M = Mazes. From Bracken and McCallum, 1998.

designed to be culturally fair. The examiner should describe the student's comfort level with the materials. The UNIT includes line drawings and objects that are recognizable to individuals from most cultures, but it may be apparent to the examiner that a particular student is puzzled by certain stimuli. This information is important to note.

Fourth, because the UNIT offers three batteries to choose from, the Abbreviated Battery, the Standard Battery, and the Extended Battery—administration time can be controlled by the examiner, depending on the number of subtests administered. The examiner should describe in the psychological report the reason for the examination and the rationale for choosing a particular version of the test. Obviously, the greatest amount of information is gained by using the Extended Battery. Therefore, when the intent is to obtain as much diagnostic information as possible, the Extended Battery should be administered. The two-subtest Abbreviated Battery offers the least information, but it consists of two psychometrically strong subtests and serves as an excellent intellectual screener. The Standard Battery offers both diagnostic information and a very good measure of g. We anticipate that the four-subtest Standard Battery will be used routinely for educational decision-making.

Summary of Interpretive Steps

The guidelines for conducting steps 2 through 6 can be summarized by adhering to the procedures described below. These procedures are most amenable to interpreting the Extended Battery; guidelines for interpreting the Standard and Abbreviated Batteries follow. (See Appendix A for a summary of the steps.)

The Test Model interpretive process relies on interpreting a multidimensional test according to the theoretical model that underpins the development of the test. For example, based on his clinical experience, Wechsler believed that human cognitive performance could be categorized parsimoniously into a dichotomous verbal/nonverbal fashion (Wechsler, 1939). For some children such a dichotomy works well, and the rational-intuitive model explains their cognitive functioning accurately. Similarly, the UNIT reasoning/memory or symbolic/nonsymbolic dichotomies may provide a parsimonious explanation for some examinees' intellectual abilities. However, in other cases neither the UNIT reasoning/memory nor the symbolic/nonsymbolic dichotomy fully explains the examinee's abilities. In such cases, the application of other theoretical orientations may be helpful for understanding the student's abilities; alternative models can be investigated as well.

- The two primary UNIT scales are Reasoning and Memory. Examiners should first consider the two primary scales that define these two factors (i.e., Memory, Reasoning) before examining the two secondary scales (i.e., Symbolic, Nonsymbolic). Hypotheses for interpreting memory/reasoning strengths and weaknesses are in Tables 3.2 through 3.5, as taken from the *UNIT Manual.*

- Consistent with steps 2 and 3, contrast the Memory Quotient with the Reasoning Quotient by subtracting one quotient from the other and examining Rapid Reference 3.12 and 3.13 to determine whether the resulting score difference is statistically significant and abnormally large, respectively. If so, this difference should be interpreted in step 4. You must use a difference score of 20 or larger to meet the criterion for "abnormally large." Remember, if considerable scatter exists among subtests *within* a scale, the affected scales may not be representative of the intended ability (e.g., reasoning); subtest scatter can be investigated in step 5.

- Also consistent with steps 2 and 3, contrast the Symbolic Quotient with the Nonsymbolic Quotient by subtracting one quotient from the other, and by examining the values in Rapid Reference 3.12 to determine whether the resulting score difference is significant. Refer to Rapid Reference 3.13 (or use our suggestion of a 20-point difference) to determine whether an abnormally large difference exists. If differences among the global scales exist, interpret those in step 4. If not, go on to step 5. See Tables 3.4 and 3.5 for hypotheses associated with strengths and weaknesses in symbolic and nonsymbolic processing.

- Consistent with step 5, examine subtest strengths and weaknesses. Subtest scores can be compared to their scale mean (e.g., memory) or the mean of the entire test. If there are statistically significant and abnormally large difference between scales, and the scatter within scales is not abnormally large, scale means should be used. If not, the overall or "pooled" mean should be used. Any subtest that deviates from the mean significantly ($p < .05$) should be considered either a strength or a weakness (see Rapid Reference 3.14). Use task analysis to determine

subtest abilities and consider the unique skills that underlie each identified subtest in Table 3.3. Reconcile any apparent inconsistencies that
might exist. Obviously, abilities measured by subtests that are designated as strengths should be eliminated as strengths if they are also assessed by other subtests as weaknesses. Remember to check subtest
specificities in Rapid Reference 3.15. Determine the relevance of intra-subtest scatter characteristics. For example, some examinees fail
easy items but pass more difficult ones, which may be indicative of educational problems such as attentional deficits or learning disabilities.
Consider educational and psychological ramifications of identified
strengths and weaknesses (e.g., high memory/low reasoning).

- Consider intervention strategies that might remediate or accommodate identified weaknesses. When possible, the examiner should link
the test results to specific to-be-learned classroom skills (e.g., calculation of addition problems) rather than attempt to remediate hypothetical constructs such as "reasoning" or "memory."

- Determine how the success of proposed intervention strategies can
best be evaluated.

Assumptions Underlying Interpretation

Systematic interpretation of UNIT scores is based on several assumptions, as
discussed by its authors. These assumptions are important because, once accepted, they prescribe the logic of the interpretive process. First, the authors
believe that intelligence is best treated as a pervasive attribute for most individuals (e.g., general intellectual ability or g factor); of course, individuals who
have suffered head trauma, brain damage or disease, or who have an unusual
central nervous system may show extreme variability in their specific intellectual abilities. Even among intact and healthy individuals there may exist considerable variability in cognitive strengths and weaknesses. Consequently, the
first assumption is that intelligence is best characterized by a hierarchical
model that has general intellectual ability, or g, at the apex, with a modest number of primary abilities and many secondary abilities that collectively comprise
g. Because the essence of intelligence is pervasive and highly generalizable, it
encompasses nearly all activities and actions and it applies fairly robustly to
multiple settings and tasks.

The second assumption suggests that sound test interpretation can be conducted only when tests possess reasonably good psychometric properties. Bracken (1987) recommended basic rules of thumb for acceptable psychometric criteria. For example, global scores used for making placement decisions should evidence reliability at a level of .90 or better; scores used for screening purposes should have reliability at a level of .80 or better. Also, item gradients should be sufficiently sensitive to capture small differences in actual ability. In addition, subtest specificity data must meet commonly accepted criteria before subtests can be considered as measures of unique abilities or skills.

All subtests within an instrument contribute to the measurement of general cognitive ability, as well as specific cognitive skills or abilities. For example, the Cube Design subtest assesses reasoning, but, it also assesses some unique ability not assessed by any other subtest. According to Kaufman (1979), if a subtest's unique variance exceeds 25% of the subtest's total variance and if its unique variance is greater than its error variance, the subtest can be interpreted as measuring some unique ability in addition to its contribution to subscale and full scale scores. See Rapid Reference 3.14 for subtest characteristics, including specificity, reliability, g loadings, and error.

The third, and perhaps most important assumption about test interpretation requires that subtest interpretation should not be conducted merely by examining test scores; any hypotheses generated from subtest analyses should be considered tentative and should be subject to verification by extra-test data (e.g., behavioral observations, work samples, third-party reports).

Current practice and state regulations dictate that intelligence tests scores not be used in isolation. Critics such as McDermott et al. (1990) have failed to examine the clinical value of subtest analysis when it is employed as only one bit of data that is confirmed or refuted through other data sources. Thus, we recommend that UNIT subtest analysis be conducted to generate hypotheses about children's unique intellectual strengths and weaknesses, but never without additional extra-test information that will allow the examiner to further evaluate the hypotheses that are generated.

The fourth assumption that underlies UNIT interpretation posits that the UNIT is a sound measure of general intelligence. Jensen (1980) concluded that many measures used to assess intelligence perform reasonably well for that purpose. According to Jensen, intelligence can be defined as the g factor, or first unrotated factor, of an indefinitely large and varied battery of mental tests.

≡Rapid Reference 3.15

Subtest Reliabilities, *g* Loadings, Specificities, and Error

| Subtest | Reliability | g Loading | | Subtest Specificity % | Error % |
		Standard Battery	Extended Battery		
Symbolic Memory	.85	.74	.73	32	15
Cube Design	.91	.78	.73	37	9
Spatial Memory	.81	.79	.77	21	19
Analogic Reasoning	.79	.74	.73	26	21
Object Memory	.76	NA	.71	26	24
Mazes	.64	NA	.44	45	36

Further, he defined "mental" capacities as those that produce individual variation in the population, other than sensory or motor abilities. According to Jensen, a task measures *g* as a function of task complexity. Any kind of task may measure *g* just as well as any type of task. The capacity of a wide variety of tasks to assess *g* has been referred to by Spearman (1927) as the principle of the "indifference of the indicator." We believe that it is possible to assess *g* as well as primary intellectual abilities (e.g., memory, reasoning) through nonverbal assessment procedures, and that the UNIT subtests are sound measures of *g*. In fact, five of the six subtests can be considered "good" measures of *g* using Kaufman's (1999) criterion of .70 and above (see Rapid Reference 3.15 for *g* loadings and 3.16 for a summary of the assumptions associated with UNIT interpretation).

Interpretation of the Standard Battery

The four-subtest Standard Battery lends itself to interpretation using the same strategies outlined for the Extended Battery, with minor modifications. As with the Extended Battery, it is most appropriate to progress in interpretation from global scores to the most specific scores. Examiners should interpret all composite scores relative to normative data, then use a systematic strategy for the subtest interpretation. However, because the Standard Battery contains only four subtests, the extent of possible subtest interpretation is limited. The examiner can and should contrast the Memory Quotient with the Reasoning Quotient, and the Symbolic Quotient with the Nonsymbolic Quotient. Within-scale variability can be investigated in a paired comparison fashion by contrasting one subtest with another. The following guidelines provide specific details for interpreting the Standard Battery.

≡Rapid Reference 3.16

Assumptions Underlying UNIT Interpretation

1. Intelligence is best understood as a general pervasive ability; thus interpretation should begin by examining global scores first.

2. Sound interpretation is based on sound psychometric and technical properties.

3. Hypotheses obtained by examining test scores should be verified by extra-test data.

4. The UNIT is a sound measure of intelligence, even though it is administered nonverbally, as determined by examination of test development characteristics, psychometric properties, and results of various special validity studies.

1. The UNIT FSIQ should be described quantitatively and qualitatively (e.g., standard score, confidence interval, percentile rank, classification of intellectual range).

2. The UNIT scale scores (i.e., Reasoning Scale, Memory Scale, Symbolic Scale, Nonsymbolic Scale) should be contrasted next, in order to examine variability across scales. If there are no significant and abnormally large differences among the UNIT scales, the FSIQ can be described as a good index of the examinee's overall cognitive ability. If one or both scales show significant and abnormally large differences, the FSIQ may be described as a poor representation of

the child's overall intellectual ability. In this case, pair-wise subtest comparisons can be made using a difference of 5 points as the criterion to establish a statistically significant and abnormally large difference.

3. If there are no significant discrepancies among scales, the examiner may wish to use the pooled procedure to determine whether subtests differ significantly from the overall subtest mean; however, typically there will be little subtest variability in this situation. Use Rapid Reference 3.14 to determine the value required to establish whether particular subtests indicate relative strengths or weaknesses. Subtest specificity must be considered from Rapid Reference 3.15 before interpreting individual subtests as measures of unique abilities. Assuming sufficient specific variance, abilities that underlie each subtest can be obtained from Table 3.3 to assist in identifying why the examinee demonstrated a strength or weakness on that particular subtest. Individual strengths and weaknesses should be cross-referenced to rule out conflicting findings and contradictory interpretations. That is, the examiner should ensure that abilities cited as strengths are not also identified elsewhere as weaknesses.

4. The last interpretive step requires that intra-subtest scatter be examined. The pattern of correct versus incorrect items within subtests should be considered. Instructionally relevant diagnostic and prescriptive information may be obtained in this manner. For example, children who have attention deficits may miss easy items due to inattention, yet correctly complete more difficult items.

Interpretation of the Abbreviated Battery

The two-subtest Abbreviated Battery provides a good measure of g, and it has good psychometric properties. The two subtests included on the Abbreviated Battery are among the strongest subtests, that is, they have excellent psychometric qualities. The following steps are suggested for interpreting the Abbreviated Battery.

1. Interpret the Abbreviated Battery Full Scale Intelligence Quotient (FSIQ) in context. That is, obtain percentile ranks, confidence interval, and intelligence classification for the FSIQ.

2. The Abbreviated Battery provides a reasonable estimate of an examinee's overall intellectual functioning. The use of one memory subtest (i.e., Symbolic Memory) and one reasoning subtest (i.e., Cube Design) limits interpretation largely to the full scale score. It is possible, however, to compare Symbolic Memory with Cube Design to infer a memory/reasoning difference in abilities. If the difference is greater than five points it can be considered large enough to be both "nonchance" and "rare." If such a difference exists, it may be useful to consider what that difference might mean. A reasonable hypothesis would be that the Symbolic Memory subtest is influenced by memory more than any other ability and that Cube Design is influenced by reasoning more than any other ability. Thus, the difference would be attributed to differences in memory and reasoning abilities. A second hypothesis might be related to symbolic (i.e., Symbolic Memory) versus nonsymbolic (i.e., Cube Design) processing, or an interaction between the abilities assessed by the primary and secondary scales.

3. Examine subtest performance for intra-subtest variability (i.e., item response patterns). Consider that item variability may be related to attentional problems, learning disabilities, or other conditions.

SUMMARY

Chapter 3 focuses on introducing multidimensional nonverbal tests of intelligence and on the administration, scoring, and interpretation of the UNIT. The UNIT is one of two nonverbal multidimensional tests available. Chapters 5 and 6 describe the other multidimensional nonverbal test, the Leiter International Performance Scale–Revised. The bulk of Chapter 3 is devoted to describing in detail information examiners need to use the test effectively, including the completely nonverbal administration procedures, scoring criteria, and extensive interpretation guidelines. Effective use of the UNIT will come from reading the *UNIT Manual,* this chapter, and Chapter 4 (Multidimensional Tests: Strengths and Weaknesses of the UNIT).

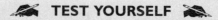

TEST YOURSELF

1. **Which one of the following subtests is included on the Reasoning Scale?**
   (a) Object Memory
   (b) Photo Series
   (c) Cube Design
   (d) Object Assembly

2. **The UNIT is based on what theory?**
   (a) Jensen's Level I (memory) and II (reasoning), with g at the apex
   (b) Cattel-Horn's Gf-Gc
   (c) Thurstone's Primary Abilities
   (d) Gardner's Multiple Intelligences

3. **Which test was standardized using NO language?**
   (a) Leiter-R
   (b) Columbia
   (c) WISC-III Performance Scale
   (d) UNIT

4. **Which two subtests are *not* included as part of the UNIT Standard Battery?**
   (a) Mazes and Cube Design
   (b) Mazes and Symbolic Reasoning
   (c) Object Memory and Cube Design
   (d) Object Memory and Mazes

5. **An abnormally large discrepancy between MQ and RQ means the discrepancy is**
   (a) Rare among the population
   (b) At least a 30-point discrepancy
   (c) At least a 5-point discrepancy
   (d) Equivalent to a statistically significant discrepancy

6. **The UNIT yields which of the following Global Scores?**
   (a) Auditory Quotient
   (b) Visual Quotient
   (c) Reasoning Quotient
   (d) Long-term Memory Quotient

7. Which of the UNIT subtests require working under time constraints?

(a) Cube Design and Mazes

(b) Symbolic Memory and Cube Design

(c) Mazes and Object Memory

(d) Spatial Memory and Mazes

8. Examiners may talk during administration of the UNIT in order to

(a) Administer the Mazes subtest

(b) Administer the Cube Design subtest

(c) Establish rapport

(d) Obtain an explanation for item failures

9. Which of the UNIT subtests produces the poorest psychometric qualities?

(a) Cube Design

(b) Symbolic Memory

(c) Object Memory

(d) Mazes

10. Performance on which one of the UNIT global scales is assumed to be most amenable to verbal mediation?

(a) Memory

(b) Reasoning

(c) Symbolic

(d) Nonsymbolic

Answers: 1. c; 2. a; 3. d; 4. d; 5. a; 6. c; 7. a; 8. c; 9. d; 10. c

Four

The UNIT provides a relatively comprehensive and user-friendly assessment of intelligence. It is designed to be completely nonverbal, and it is the only multidimensional test that offers 100% nonverbal administration, using demonstration and sample items, gestures, and pantomime. The test offers a number of strengths. However, as with all tests, it is not perfect. The UNIT has some salient weaknesses as well. Even though the test was published recently, two independent reviews are already available (Fachting & Bradley-Johnson, in press; Fives & Flanagan, 2000). In addition, we have had an opportunity to evaluate the test during its development, to use the test for about one year, and to obtain feedback from our students and from professionals all over the country who use the test. Consequently, we have considerable information regarding the test's pros and cons. For example, we know that a strong, representative standardization sample was obtained, that the test is easy to administer and score, and that the authors and publisher worked very hard to ensure fairness for all examinees. Also, we are aware of some weaknesses, including a less-than-optimal floor for the Abbreviated Battery for very young, cognitively delayed individuals, and a standardization sample that includes only school-age examinees.

Independent reviews have generally been favorable. Fachting and Bradley-Johnson (in press) conclude their review by noting that the UNIT is a welcome addition to present methods of measuring intellectual functioning in a nonvocal manner. Fives and Flanagan (2000) conclude by noting that the UNIT "is theoretically driven . . . psychometrically sound . . . and appears to be highly useful." They also point out several specific advantages, including the completely nonverbal administration; the ability to measure multiple abilities; the inclusion of Abbreviated, Standard, and Extended Battery forms; the comprehensiveness of the normative sample; the ability to distinguish between abstract tasks and those that require the use of internal verbal mediation; and an "exemplary" record form. Other specific strengths (and some limitations) are pointed out by both sets of reviewers and we mention some of those below, along with others we consider important. We have grouped the strengths and weaknesses into the following categories: test development, administration and scoring, standardization, reliability and validity, and interpretation (also see Rapid References 4.1, 4.2, 4.3, 4.4, and 4.5). We follow the discussion of strengths and weaknesses by mentioning several test development characteristics designed to ensure fairness.

TEST DEVELOPMENT STRENGTHS

A fundamental strength of the UNIT is its strong theoretical base, consistent with the models of Carroll (1993) and Jensen (1980), both of whom consider intelligence to be hierarchically structured and multifaceted. Bracken and McCallum (1998) define intelligence as "the ability to problem solve using memory and reasoning" (p. 12). Thus, the model posits a multifaceted arrangement with general intelligence at the apex and the two broad but subordinate factors of memory and reasoning at a level just below g. Subordinate to the primary factors of memory and reasoning are the secondary factors of symbolic and nonsymbolic (covert) mediation. The model represents a strength for two basic reasons. First, a wealth of research supports the hierarchical nature of intelligence and the importance of memory and reasoning as basic building blocks (see Bracken & McCallum, 1998; Jensen, 1980). Second, as Fives and Flanagan (2000) point out, the UNIT is unique in that its underlying theory is both correlational and experimental. Both correlational (e.g., factor analyses) and experimental (e.g., lab manipulation) methodologies were instrumental in producing the support literature for the UNIT. That is, from the correlational literature we know that successful problem solving requires application of memory and reasoning; from the experimental literature we know that the processing strategies relying on symbolic and nonsymbolic mediation are critical. Others have noted the importance of categorizing theories or models of intelligence based on their methodological origins (e.g., Sternberg & Powell, 1982).

Development of the UNIT was guided by 10 research and development goals; these goals are described in the *UNIT Manual* and are reproduced in Rapid Reference 3.2. Some of the more salient goals include: to ensure fairness by eliminating or reducing sources of bias, to encourage efficient administration by including three formats, to ensure 100% nonverbal administration, to assess intelligence with psychometric rigor, and to incorporate tasks that maximize examiner knowledge and experience. Similarly, the authors adopted a list of 10 item selection criteria (see the *UNIT Manual* for elaboration). Those criteria require that: item presentation must be entirely nonverbal; item responses must be entirely nonverbal; task demands must be communicated easily through physical gestures, demonstration, sample, and checkpoint items; nonverbal stimuli (e.g., gestures) must be familiar to individuals from dominant world cultures; speeded responding must be deemphasized; items must be visually stimulating and interesting in order to elicit active participation; items must be sensitive to differences of gender, ethnicity, and race; item presentation must be brief, simple, and clear; and items must reflect the theoretical orientation of the subtest (recall of symbolic stimuli). See Rapid Reference 4.1 for specific strengths and weaknesses.

STRENGTHS AND WEAKNESSES OF ADMINISTRATION AND SCORING

The *UNIT Manual* contains details of administration and scoring; in addition, an 8½ × 11 inch laminated card called "Administration at a Glance" provides abbreviated directions and a description of the eight gestures used during standardization. In addition, as the *Manual* suggests, even though the test is nonverbal the examiner and examinee can communicate through a common language (or a translator), and should. The test administration should not be silent and stilted. Examiners should use a common language to establish rapport, discuss the examinee's history, and so forth as is useful. The examiner can and should talk, just not about the UNIT task demands.

Several innovative administrative and scoring characteristics aid the examination process. Fives and Flanagan (2000) note some of the innovations, observing that they include a "scoring procedure for the Mazes . . . clearly superior and more user friendly than the Mazes subtest of the WISC-III. "Moreover, they note that most tests include three traditional item types (i.e., sample, demonstration, and scored items), but that the UNIT includes a fourth type, called "checkpoint," to ensure maintenance of the desired response set. Checkpoint items are scored, but the examiner may provide feedback if the examinee fails these items. These items help ensure that the examinee understands the task demands.

The UNIT offers three administration formats: an Abbreviated Battery, a

≡Rapid Reference 4.1

Strengths and Weaknesses of UNIT Development

Strengths

- Subtest selection was guided by 10 research and development guidelines (see Rapid Reference 3.2).
- Item selection was guided by 10 selection criteria, as reported on pages 17 and 18 of the UNIT Manual, and summarized above.
- Thirteen fairness criteria were observed in developing the UNIT (see Rapid Reference 4.7 for a complete list). They include elimination of language from test administration, limited influence of speed, and use of ample teaching items (for elaboration, see McCallum, 1999).
- Several of the subtests make use of existing subtest formats to ensure user-friendliness (positive transfer) for examiners.
- Subtests allow use of creative administration and scoring procedures to increase floors, ceilings, and variability; consequently, it is possible to administer the same subtests across the entire age range.

Weaknesses

- The age range extends from 5 years to 17 years 11 months only.
- The artwork for Matrix Analogies and Object Memory contain black and white line drawings only and may not be maximally engaging for young children.

Standard Battery, and an Extended Battery. These formats allow for administration of two, four, and six subtests, respectively, requiring from 15 to 45 minutes to administer. The record book is clear and inclusive; it offers start and stop rules, correct responses, and other useful information, including an inclusive worksheet for subtest interpretation. To facilitate learning to administer the UNIT, Riverside publishing company offers a video tape and a CD showing administration of the test, a *University Training Guide* (Bracken & McCallum, 1999), and a computer scoring/interpretation program to be released in 2001.

Fives and Flanagan (2000) point out a couple of administration limitations. They note that the administration directions are printed in the *Manual* and on the Administration at a Glance card rather than on the easel, and consequently may not be as user-friendly for those familiar with easel-based directions. They also note that administration may begin at either end of the easel and move in either direction, which may be confusing to some examiners. That is, items are printed on both sides of each page. However, to prevent confusion, the careful examiner will note that the easel cover lists in green the subtests that can be administered in a particular direction; in addition, green tabs are used to orient the examiner. Other specific administration and scoring strengths and weaknesses are shown in Rapid Reference 4.2.

STRENGTHS AND WEAKNESSES OF UNIT TECHNICAL PROPERTIES

The *UNIT Manual* provides a wealth of reliability and validity data. Two types of reliability data are presented—internal and test-retest. In addition, both internal and external validity data are reported. Age-related growth curves and results from exploratory and confirmatory factor analyses are shown as evidence of internal validity. Correlations with other measures of intelligence and various measures of achievement provide evidence of external validity. Item gradient and floor/ceiling data are shown as well.

Internal consistency reliability indices are .91 and above for all the Full Scale IQs across all batteries. Composite (scale) scores range from .86 to .91 for the Standard Battery. As might be expected, subtest reliabilities are lower, ranging from .64 (Mazes) to .91 (Cube Design). Subtests on the Standard Battery range from .79 (Analogic Reasoning) to .91 (Cube Design). Fives and Flanagan (2000) conclude that the "effectiveness of the UNIT in this domain is further illustrated by the high levels of internal consistency when the instrument is used for clinical populations typically found in the clinical settings." The UNIT reports consistently high reliabilities for the combined clinical populations taken from the various validity studies (e.g., .92 for the FSIQ). Split-half reliabilities are less impressive, ranging from .58 (Mazes) to .85 (Cube Design); again, the subtests in the Standard Battery yield more impressive values, though they range from only .68 (Spatial Memory) to .85 (Cube Design).

Content/construct validity was determined in part by examining growth

Rapid Reference 4.2

Strengths and Weaknesses of UNIT Administration and Scoring

Strengths

- The UNIT offers 100% nonverbal subtest administration and is the only multidimensional nonverbal test standardized with absolutely no language; however, the examiner can talk to the examinee to establish and maintain rapport if they have a common language.

- The record form is very user-friendly, and includes salient starting/stopping rules and correct answers; it also includes descriptive classifications built into the profile sheet.

- There are three administration formats (batteries) depending on available time and need; the Abbreviated Battery contains two subtests and is useful for screening, the Standard Battery contains four subtests and is useful for providing scores for most routine placement decisions, and the Extended Battery contains six subtests and is most useful for providing additional diagnostic information.

- The *Manual* offers extremely detailed administration directions; in addition, each kit comes with an 8½ × 11 inch laminated "Administration at a Glance" sheet with abbreviated directions. This sheet also contains a picture of each of the eight administration gestures and a brief description of the three administration formats. Standard scores, percentiles, and SEm values are found on one page.

Weaknesses

- Administration is completely nonverbal, and may seem awkward initially. The examiner must master use of the eight gestures. The examiner may talk, but cannot talk about the subtest demands.

- The Mazes are not scored dichotomously, so scoring is different than on subtests using more conventional scoring strategies. Administration of the Mazes requires that the examiner stop the child at the point of the first error; the first incorrect decision point in the maze. Each correct decision point is scored one point, so the examiner must attend to the templates shown on the Record Booklet during this subtest.

- The directions are found in the *Manual* and on the Administration at a Glance card, not on the easel. Thus, for examiners familiar with the other tests that use easel-based directions, administration may initially seem more cumbersome.

- The easel containing the Standard Battery allows administration in both directions. That is, the pages contain items front and back, and may initially confuse the examiner. The examiner should note that the front of the easel shows in green the name of each of the two subtests appropriate for that particular direction.

(continued)

Strengths

- With the exception of the manipulatives (e.g., blocks, chips, pencils) stimulus materials are presented in two user-friendly easels. The first easel contains materials for the Standard Battery, and the second for the Object Memory subtest.

- Scoring rules and reverse rules are consistently applied.

- Exposure times for the stimulus plates on the memory subtests are the same across the three memory subtests.

- The *Manual* includes figures showing the appropriate arrangement of test materials, examiner, and examinee for every subtest.

- The *Manual* shows clearly the eight gestures used in the standardization of the UNIT.

- There are several media products available that demonstrate and describe administration of the subtests, including a traditional VCR tape, a CD-Rom, and a convenient 67-page *University Training Manual*. In addition, a computer scoring and interpretation program will be available in 2001.

- The examinee uses chips to mark the chosen cells on the Spatial Memory subtest, reducing examiner scoring error.

- With the exception of the Block Design and the Mazes subtests, scoring is dichotomous.

Weaknesses

curves. Children become more cognitively sophisticated as they age; hence, their raw scores should increase with age. W-scores growth curves maintain the age-dependent relationship between cognitive sophistication and age, and the *UNIT Manual* shows consistent W-score gains on all subtests as a function of age. Additional indices of internal validity were obtained using exploratory and confirmatory factor analyses. Support for the hierarchical structure of the UNIT, with *g* at the apex, is provided by results from both principal components and principal axis methods of extraction. Using an oblique rotation, an eigen value of 2.33 was obtained for the first factor and .64 for the second, indicating strong support for *g*. Additional analyses also show support for the two-factor memory/reasoning structure, with subtests assigned to the memory factor loading significantly on that factor, and subtests assigned to the reasoning factor loading on it. Second-order analyses provided similar results, showing strong first-order memory and reasoning factors in addition to a higher order *g* factor. Additional exploratory and confirmatory procedures provided support for the overall structure, showing evidence in support of *g,* memory, and reasoning, and the lower-order symbolic and nonsymbolic factors. Multiple goodness of fit statistics are provided using the confirmatory procedures.

Floor and ceiling data are shown in detail in the *Manual* and exhibit good properties in general; however, the floor is somewhat limited for very young (5-year-old) examinees who exhibit delayed cognitive abilities. In fact, the Abbreviated Battery is not recommended for seriously cognitively delayed 5-year-old examinees for this reason. The lowest possible FSIQ score for a 5-year-old child on the Abbreviated Battery is 72. Fachting and Bradley-Johnson (in press) recommend that low scores on the Abbreviated Battery should be interpreted carefully and examined further with other intellectual measures for the youngest children. The floor is much less limited for the Standard and Extended Batteries. For example, the lowest scores possible for a 5-year-old on those batteries are 61 and 54, respectively. UNIT ceilings are excellent for the oldest examinees; the highest possible FSIQs for the oldest examinees exceed three standard deviations above the mean for all batteries.

Item gradients are good, and as Fives and Flanagan (2000) note, care was taken to ensure that correct performance on each item changed the examinee's scaled score by no more than .33 standard deviation. Extensive item gradient and floor/ceiling tables are presented in the *Manual* for the examiner's convenience. See Rapid Reference 4.3 for technical strengths and weaknesses.

Rapid Reference 4.3

Strengths and Weaknesses of UNIT Technical Properties

Strengths

- Actual obtained correlation coefficients and those corrected for restriction and expansion in range using Gulliksen's (1987) formula are reported in the UNIT Manual.

- Split-half reliability coefficients and standard errors of measurement are excellent for the global scores, including the Full Scale IQ, Reasoning Quotient, Memory Quotient, Symbolic Quotient, and Nonsymbolic Quotient. For example, the average reliability across all ages from the standardization sample for the FSIQ is .93 for the Standard and Extended Batteries and .91 for the Abbreviated Battery.

- Across all 12 age groups, 83% of the subtests yielded reliability coefficients about 80 (Standard Battery), and the average across all ages ranged from .79 (Analogic Reasoning) to .91 (Cube Design).

- In addition to providing reliability coefficients for the standardization sample data, coefficients are also provided for a clinical/exceptional sample; across all subtest and global scores the average reliabilities for this example exceed .90, with one exception: the Mazes subtest yielded a reliability estimate of .82.

- Reliability coefficients are also provided at two critical decision-making points for FSIQs (i.e., 70 and 130), a first for any test as far as we know. For the Extended Battery, obtained r for the global scores ranged from .83 to .90; corrected r (for restriction in range) ranged from .95 to .98. For the Standard Battery, obtained r ranged from .79 to .91; corrected r ranged from .96 to .98.

- Practice effects are reported and range from +4.8 (Extended Battery) to +7.2 (Abbreviated Battery) over approximately 3 weeks. Gains in the Standard and Extended FSIQs average about three to five points over the test-retest interval.

Weaknesses

- Some subtests yielded average subtest reliabilities below .80 (i.e., split-half reliabilities are .76 and .64 for Object Memory and Mazes, respectively; test-retest values for five of the six subtests are below .80).

- Test-retest reliability coefficients are reported for four age groups and the total sample and are generally below the split-half values; for the total sample, global score obtained coefficients ranged from .74 to .84 for the Standard Battery and .75 to .81 for the Extended Battery. Corrected coefficients ranged from .78 to .88 for the Standard Battery and from .79 to .85 for the Extended Battery. The Abbreviated Battery yielded obtained and corrected r values of .79 and .83, respectively.

- The specific variance for Spatial Memory, though greater than error variance, is less than 25%, making it less interpretable as a measure of a unique cognitive ability—though not a strong measure of memory.

- Because the floor is limited for cognitively limited 5-year old examinees for the Abbreviated Battery, we recommend that examiners not use the Abbreviated Battery with children of this age suspected of having mental retardation.

Strengths

- Exploratory and confirmatory factor analyses yield support for the UNIT theoretical model. Five of six subtests yield a *g* loading of .71 or better; a value considered good by Kaufman (1999); these values support the assertion that the UNIT provides a sound measure of *g*. In addition, the *Manual* reports confirmatory factor analytic data showing support for the Memory–Reasoning and Symbolic–Nonsymbolic organizational arrangement.

- The *UNIT Manual* reports results of a number of concurrent validity studies with various measures of intelligence for different populations. Correlation coefficients showing the relationship between UNIT FSIQs and full scale scores from other major intelligence tests (e.g., Wechsler scales, Woodcock-Johnson Cognitive Battery) are typically in the .70 to .80 range. Coefficients between the UNIT FSIQs and three nonverbal measures (i.e., Matrix Analogies Test, Test of Nonverbal Intelligence-2, and the Raven's Standard Progressive Matrices test) are typically in the .60 to .80 range.

- The *UNIT Manual* reports correlations between UNIT scores and those from a variety of achievement tests; coefficients typically range from .20 to .50 between global UNIT scores and various achievement scores from tests such as the Peabody Individual Achievement Test-Revised (Dunn & Dunn, 1981), Wechsler Individual Achievement Test (Wechsler, 1991), and the Woodcock Johnson-Revised, Achievement Battery (Woodcock & Johnson, 1989/1990). Obtained and corrected coefficients are reported.

- Consistent with predictions from the UNIT theoretical model, coefficients between the Symbolic Quotient and various verbal and achievement measures are typically higher than the coefficients between the Nonsymbolic Quotient and verbal/achievement measures. In fact, about two-thirds of the relationships show higher Symbolic Quotient—verbal/achievement coefficients.

- Specific variance values are sufficient for all subtests except Spatial Memory; thus, with the exception of this subtest, all can be interpreted on their own, that is, as measures of unique abilities.

Weaknesses

STRENGTHS AND WEAKNESSES OF THE UNIT STANDARDIZATION

Standardization data were collected from 108 sites in 38 states; the sample included 2,100 children and adolescents ranging in age from 5 years 0 months to 17 years 11 months and 30 days.

The data were collected based on a stratified random selection procedure and is representative of the 1995 census data (U.S. Bureau of the Census, 1995) and of the school age population. To ensure adequate sampling of regular and special needs children, authors included representative samples of children from various special education categories according to figures taken from a variety of sources, including the *Seventeenth Annual Report to Congress on the Implementation of the Individuals with Disabilities Education Act* (IDEA; U.S. Department of Education, 1995). The following stratification variables were included: sex, race, Hispanic origin, region, community setting, classroom placement, special education services, and parental educational attainment. Special school populations, based on exceptionality, included children with learning disabilities (5.6% of the UNIT sample, 5.9% of the population), speech and language impairments (2.3%, 2.4%), emotional disturbance (0.9%, 1.0%), mental retardation (1.2%, 1.3%), hearing impairments (0.2%, 0.2%), intellectual giftedness (6.2%, 6.4%), bilingual education (1.8%, 3.1%), and English as a second language (2.0%, 4.0%).

For standardization, examiners were screened based on their training and experience administering standardized tests. Selected examiners were provided additional specialized training using a videotape at training sites around the country. During training and standardization each completed protocol was checked against 33 criteria and those considered suspect were examined and either "passed" after clarification from the examiner, or eliminated. Specific strengths and weaknesses are shown in Rapid Reference 4.4.

STRENGTHS AND WEAKNESSES OF UNIT INTERPRETATION

The *UNIT Manual* provides a wealth of information examiners will find useful for interpretation. Guidelines are provided for normative and ipsative interpretation, along with an extensive number of tables showing step-by-step strategies for hypothesis generation. Examinees are encouraged to begin the

≡ Rapid Reference 4.4

Strengths and Weaknesses of the UNIT Standardization

Strengths

- The standardization sample was well stratified on the key variables, including, sex, race, Hispanic origin, region, community setting, classroom placement, parental educational attainment, and school-based special needs category.
- Normative data were obtained from 2,100 children; an additional 1,765 children and adolescents participated in the reliability, validity, and fairness studies.
- Data were collected from 108 sites in 38 states.
- Standardization data (e.g., test booklets) were subjected to a 33-point quality control procedure.

Weaknesses

- Standardization data were collected for school-age children only.
- Although the percentages of special education students in the population match closely the percentages in the UNIT sample, the bilingual and ESL samples were underrepresented slightly (1.8% in sample, 3.1% in the population for the bilingual sample; 2% versus 4% for the ESL sample).

interpretation process by focusing on normative comparisons, taking into account test error. Interpretation should proceed from the general to the specific, from the molar to the molecular; that is, examination should begin by focusing on the most global scores (i.e., scale scores), followed by examination of subtest scores. Finally, examiners should focus on item performance and even on specific problem solving attack strategies using a qualitative approach. UNIT authors acknowledge the controversy surrounding the practice of ipsative interpretation, but recommend the procedure, noting that ipsative test data should be used cautiously. For example, test data can be used to generate hypotheses; these data should be used as part of a larger knowledge network characterizing the individual—never in isolation. Hypotheses should be checked against extra-test data.

In addition to tables showing suggested interpretative hypotheses, the

UNIT Manual provides many others to aid in the interpretative process. For example, there are tables showing abilities assumed to underlie subtest performance, test-age equivalents, floor/ceiling and item gradient data, subtest technical properties, base rates, and levels of statistical significance corresponding to various differences between subtest and scaled scores.

Interpretation of the UNIT is made relatively simple because the subtests are assigned to conceptual categories (e.g., reasoning, symbolic processing) and the authors provide straightforward interpretative guidelines. In addition, though the UNIT is multidimensional, there are only six subtests to consider. Rapid Reference 4.5 shows specific strengths and weaknesses of UNIT interpretation.

FAIRNESS

A number of considerations guided UNIT authors in their efforts to make the UNIT fair for populations for whom language-loaded tests might be problematic. In fact, the *UNIT Manual* includes an entire chapter devoted to describing test development efforts to ensure fairness and the results of fairness studies. Some of the major criteria used by the authors to ensure fairness have been described already in Rapid Reference 4.1, and a complete list is presented in Rapid Reference 4.6.

As a result of implementation of the fairness criteria, a wealth of data were generated. These data show the effects of efforts to reduce bias. For example, reliability coefficients and standard errors of measures are reported for African American and Hispanic samples separately. In addition, studies show comparable technical features across sex, race, and ethnicity (e.g., factor structure and predictive capabilities). Of course, results of independent researchers will be needed to further examine fairness. Already the results of one study are encouraging. Maller (in press) shows no evidence of differential item functioning (DIF) for deaf students compared with hearing peers.

Over the past few years some writers have argued that mean IQ differences between groups reflect bias. In contrast, several experts have argued cogently that mean differences cannot be taken as evidence of bias (e.g., Jensen, 1980; Reynolds, Lowe, & Coury, 1999). However, mean differences should not be taken lightly, and when they occur bias must be ruled out by system-

⚟Rapid Reference 4.5

Strengths and Weaknesses of UNIT Interpretation

Strengths

- The *UNIT Manual* includes extensive interpretative guidelines, including information for determining strengths and weaknesses using traditional normative and ipsative (step-by-step) strategies.

- The *UNIT Manual* includes several tables presenting interpretive hypotheses (also see Tables 3.3 and 3.4 in Chapter 3).

- Underlying abilities hypothesized to influence performance are defined in the *UNIT Manual*.

- The *UNIT Manual* includes tables providing test-age equivalents, prorated sums of scale scores when a subtest is substituted, and procedures for substituting a subtest when one is spoiled.

- The *UNIT Manual* provides base rate tables for various comparisons.

- The Record Booklet offers a number of user-friendly interpretative characteristics (e.g., interpretative worksheet lends itself to ipsative and normative analyses; descriptive categories are printed on the record form).

- A computer scoring and interpretation program will be available in 2001.

Weaknesses

- There is little in the *Manual* describing base rate interpretation procedures as presented by Glutting, McDermott, and Konold (1997).

- The floors of the Symbolic Memory and Cube Design subtests are limited for cognitively delayed 5-year-old examinees.

- The interlocking design is conceptually complex. That is, subtests are assigned to more than one conceptual category. Thus, two major influences on subtest performance (i.e., memory/reasoning or symbolic/nonsymbolic processing) must be considered before more minor abilities are examined.

Rapid Reference 4.6

Criteria Used to Ensure Fairness for UNIT

- elimination of language from test administration
- assessment of multidimensional constructs
- elimination of achievement influences
- limited influence of speeded performance
- use of variable response modes
- use of ample teaching items
- use of expert panels to select items
- use of sophisticated item bias statistics to reduce content validity bias
- comparison of psychometric properties across populations
- use of sophisticated statistical techniques to reduce construct validity bias
- comparison of mean scores across various populations
- use of strategies to reduce predictive validity bias
- inclusion of children with handicapping conditions into the standardization sample

atic scrutiny of the technical quality of the test in terms of gender, race, and ethnicity. Certainly, mean differences due to contaminating or irrelevant influences should be eliminated. For example, language limitations (e.g., limited English proficiency) should not negatively influence scores on intelligence tests. In those cases where language influences performance negatively, a language-reduced or language-free test should reduce mean differences (and be fairer).

It is possible to see the positive effects of eliminating language on mean differences between members of some minority groups and their (nonminority group) peers. UNIT data illustrate this point; the *Manual* reports a number of studies showing performance of minority and culturally different groups on the UNIT (as compared to controls matched on age, sex, and parental education level). FSIQ differences ranged from 1.43 to 2.13 between Hispanics and a demographically matched comparison sample across the Abbreviated, Standard, and Extended Batteries. FSIQ differences ranged from 3.26 to 6.50

across those same batteries between Native Americans and a demographically matched comparison group. Finally, FSIQ differences ranged from 7.63 to 9.77 across these batteries between African Americans and a demographically matched comparison sample.

The mean differences between the Hispanic and African American samples and their matched comparison groups are particular salient for a couple of reasons. First, members of these two groups comprise about 25% of the total U.S. population, and their numbers are increasing rapidly. Second, the UNIT FSIQ mean differences between members of these two groups and demographically matched controls are less than often reported for language-loaded tests. For example, Prifitera, Weiss, and Saklofske (1998) report WISC-III FSIQ differences of 14.9 and 9.4 between African Americans and Whites and Hispanics and Whites, respectively. However, it should be noted that these differences do not reflect demographically matched comparisons; when the samples are matched the differences are reduced to 11.0 and 2.8. These differences are much closer to those obtained on the UNIT, but are still slightly higher, perhaps reflecting the unwanted influence of language.

In spite of the strong fairness data reported for the UNIT, some limitations remain. Although the UNIT was developed and standardized to ensure cross-cultural fairness, it was not standardized for use in foreign countries. In addition, there are no specific methodological and statistical procedures in the *UNIT Manual* detailing how it can be adapted for use in foreign countries when full-scale restandardization is not possible. (Currently, no other test offers these guidelines, either.) Because administration of the UNIT is completely nonverbal, foreign standardization in other countries will be relatively easy, requiring translation only for directions and scoring criteria.

When full-scale restandardization is not possible, other, less costly equating or adapting procedures may be implemented. First, it will be necessary to investigate the extent to which items function differently in other countries by using bias detection strategies, such as those described by Gittler and Tanzer (1998), who used a Linear Logistic Test Model (LLTM), an extension of the dichotomous Rasch Model (RM). Latent trait procedures such as LLTM may be used in conjunction with more traditional measures such as equivalence of factor structure, reliabilities, and means to determine equivalence. Assuming lack

Rapid Reference 4.7

Guidelines for Cross-Cultural Use of the UNIT

1. Using a stratified, randomly selected sample of 200 individuals from the target culture and the standardization data from the anchor culture, establish cross-cultural item equivalence using techniques such as those described by Gittler and Tanzer (1998).

2. It may be necessary to norm the test in the target culture if the items and scales show evidence of DIF, or "poor fit," as determined by the LLTM statistics and other criteria (e.g., similarity of factor structure, reliabilities, mean differences). Criteria may be liberal or conservative based on the perceived need to use the test for a particular population.

3. Establish local norms for the target culture by using the 200 individuals identified in the original sampling to:

    (a) compute mean subtest/test raw scores at four ages;

    (b) create regression formulas to predict means for all ages;

    (c) obtain raw score differences (by age) between predicted means of target sample and U.S. standardization sample;

    (d) generate adapted norm tables by adding/subtracting raw score differences as a constant in the raw-to-scaled score transformation formula;

    (e) use existing norm table to transform sums of subtest scaled scores to composite scale scores.

of item/scale congruence, a local norming may be necessary. In Rapid Reference 4.7 we present a set of guidelines describing the general steps that might be used to determine item/scale equivalence and steps to obtain efficiently local norms. These guidelines were developed and presented by McCallum and Bracken (1999).

CLINICAL APPLICATIONS OF THE UNIT

In this section we focus on the primary clinical applications of the UNIT, including: (a) assessment of examinees from different cultural backgrounds/ minority groups; (b) those with limited English proficiency; (c) those with speech/language and hearing impairments; (d) individuals with learning disabilities or mental retardation; and (e) those with emotional disorders.

Assessment of Individuals from Different Cultural Backgrounds

In general, individuals from minority groups or from different cultural backgrounds are penalized when assessed by verbally-laden measurements; typically, these individuals are less familiar with the English language. Because the UNIT allows nonverbal assessment, it is more amenable to cross-cultural and minority group assessment than are verbal measures.

As noted in the "Fairness" section above, mean differences between groups is sometimes assumed to provide an index of bias (against the lower scoring group), assuming the groups are matched on relevant variables. However, this assumption is controversial, and as Jensen (1980) notes, there is no a priori reason to assume that all groups must be equal; there are several psychometric indicators of bias (other than mean differences) that are more rigorous. However, because mean differences create a "red flag," and because the authors of the UNIT contend that it was developed to reduce the unwanted effects of language, it is important to consider those differences when they exist.

For example, Table 6.10 in the *UNIT Manual* shows that examinees from Ecuador earned mean FSIQ scores of only 5.33 and 3.26 points less than matched controls for the Standard and Extended Batteries, respectively. A sample of Hispanic examinees earned mean FSIQ scores of only 2.13 and 1.43 points less than matched controls on the Standard and Extended Batteries, respectively (Table 6.7). Native Americans earned FSIQs of 6.50 and 6.24 less than matched controls on the Standard and Extended Batteries. African Americans earned FSIQs of 8.63 and 9.77 less than matched controls on the Standard and Extended Batteries, respectively (Table 6.6). Importantly, these mean differences are less than those typically reported for minority groups on conventional verbally loaded instruments, and suggest that the UNIT is capable of eliminating some of the ill effects associated with language. Also of interest, the differences between the groups were greater on the Symbolic (SQ) than Nonsymbolic Quotients (NSQ), except for the African American comparison. The African American SQ versus NSQ differences were minuscule.

The UNIT may be very useful for evaluating minority individuals who have good nonverbal skills relative to their verbal abilities. In fact, some State Departments of Education (e.g., Tennessee) now require the use of nonverbal tests when minority group students score well, but fail to meet criteria for gifted placement using traditional verbally laden tests. The reason for this is that minority individuals, and those from certain other protected classes (e.g., low socioeconomic status), may be unfairly impacted by heavily loaded verbal tests.

Importantly, the UNIT will likely identify individuals as gifted who are different from those typically identified by verbally laden measures. Evidence for this outcome is suggested by mean score differences between gifted examinees and nongifted matched controls reported in the *UNIT Manual*. Gifted examinees outscored nongifted examinees by 13.50 and 12.20 FSIQ points for the Standard and Extended Batteries, respectively. These differences are less than expected and indicate that many individuals who are identified as gifted using conventional verbal measures will not score as highly on the UNIT. Conversely, individuals who score very well on the UNIT may not score as well on verbal measures. Importantly, because the UNIT scores are normally distributed, they will identify approximately the same number of gifted examinees as the traditional verbally loaded measures. However, the UNIT will identify more of those individuals who have excellent nonverbal skills and fewer of those with (only) highly developed verbal abilities.

Assessment of Individuals with Limited English Proficiency

The *UNIT Manual* reports mean differences for a combined sample of bilingual/ESL examinees. These examinees earned FSIQs of 3.56 and 3.73 less than matched controls on the Standard and Extended Batteries, respectively. These individuals obviously show (English) language-related deficiencies, and consistent with this notion, the mean differences between the groups are primarily symbolic in nature (rather than nonsymbolic). These results suggest that the UNIT will be useful in assessing those with limited language facility.

Assessment of Individuals with Speech/Language and Hearing Impairments

The *UNIT Manual* reports mean differences between a sample of examinees with speech and language impairments and matched controls. Individuals with speech and language impairments earned FSIQs of 6.81 and 8.72 points less than the matched controls on the Standard and Extended Batteries, respectively. The SQ and NSQ mean score differences were approximately equal, a finding consistent with recent literature showing that many individuals with language impairments perform at lower levels relative to nonimpaired individuals on a number of cognitive tasks, including but not limited to those requiring symbolic representation ability (Montgomery, Windsor, & Stark, 1991). In fact, a common symbolic limitation associated with the ability to generate and manipulate various mental representations is assumed by some experts to underlie both linguistic *and* nonlinguistic difficulties (Montgomery et al., 1991; Savich, 1984). Consequently, it is impossible to determine whether the presence of subtle but pervasive cognitive deficits is the cause or effect of language deficits for many individuals. Even so, nonverbal measures of intelligence are typically considered more appropriate for assessing the level of cognitive functioning of those with language impairments.

Assessment of Individuals with Learning Disabilities and Mental Retardation

The *UNIT Manual* reports mean differences between individuals with learning disabilities and matched controls. Individuals with learning disabilities earned FSIQs of 10.63 and 11.03 less than matched controls on the Standard and Extended Batteries, respectively. The primary criterion associated with a diagnosis of learning disability is the presence of a discrepancy between intellectual ability and achievement, with achievement being lower. However, the magnitude of the discrepancy required for diagnosis is different in different states; in addition, other criteria must be considered, making the population highly variable. For example, the presence of scatter among scores is considered by some experts to be a critical characteristic, as is the presence of a processing deficit; in addition, there is a growing literature addressing the characteristics associated with nonverbal learning disabilities (Rourke, 1995). In short, there is considerable heterogeneity within the learning disability population, making particular predictions about score patterns difficult.

The *UNIT Manual* reports mean score differences between a sample of individuals with mental retardation and a control sample. Those with mental retardation earned FSIQs of 33.73 and 34.05 points less than matched controls on the Standard and Extended Batteries, respectively. These scores are consistent with expectations and suggest that the test is sensitive to those deficits associated with pervasive cognitive limitations.

Assessment of Individual with Emotional Disorders

The *UNIT Manual* reports mean differences between individuals with serious emotional disorders and matched controls. Those with a diagnosis of serious emotional disturbance earned mean scores of .44 and .30 points less than those in the control group for the Standard and Extended Batteries, respectively. These differences are not clinically meaningful, nor are they unexpected. Criteria required to assign a diagnosis of emotional disturbance do not require deficits in cognitive ability (see Individuals with Disabilities Education Act of 1990: IDEA-Public Law 101-476, and its 1997 reauthorization, PL 105-17).

Summary

Based on the data reported in the *UNIT Manual,* the test appears to be appropriate for individuals from a wide variety of clinical populations such as those just described. Characteristics of the UNIT make it useful for other populations as well. For example, three of the subtests (i.e., Memory subtests) require attention and good working memory. Consequently, those with attention deficits may perform poorly on those subtests, which could provide diagnostic information.

UNIT CASE STUDY

Below is a case study illustrating the interpretative steps. It is an actual case, with demographic data and background changed to ensure confidentiality.

Other examples can be found in the *UNIT Manual* (Bracken & McCallum, 1998) and the *UNIT Training Manual* (Bracken & McCallum, 1999).

Psychological Report

Name: Jon   Age: 6
School: Coffee Primary   Grade: K
Date of Birth: October 28, 1991
Parent(s)/Guardian(s) Name: Jack & Jill
Parent(s)/Guardian(s) Address:
Date(s) of Evaluation: 4/13/98, 4/28/98   Date of Report: 4/30/98

Reason for Referral

Jon was referred by his mother because he has been having difficulties at home and school. Jon's mother reported that he is overly "physical and aggressive, as well as hyperactive." Jon's kindergarten teacher reported physical aggression, as well. Additionally, he is experiencing problems making and maintaining friendships and often fails to complete school work.

Background Information

Developmental and Medical History
Jon is a 6-year-old boy who lives with his biological parents and a 3-year-old male cousin, a 4-year-old brother, and a 10-year-old brother. Jon's mother reported that the boys fight often, and that Jon sometimes bangs his head when he becomes angry or frustrated. Jon's mother reported a normal pregnancy and delivery with Jon. Although he completed developmental milestones within normal age ranges, Jon has had a history of hearing problems, which are related to chronic ear infections. Recently, tubes were surgically implanted in his ears for the second time. In addition, Jon's articulation is poor; he has difficulty enunciating certain speech sounds (e.g., the more difficult consonants and blends). Information from two observations by an educational diagnostician indicated that Jon is frequently inattentive and exhibits considerable impulsive behavior (in two settings).

Current Educational Issues and Program

Jon is currently in kindergarten and has been receiving poor grades in listening and classroom behavior. According to his mother and corroborated by his teacher, he "sometimes exhibits physically aggressive behaviors toward his peers."

Behavioral Observations

Jon accompanied the examiner to the assessment room willingly and rapport was easily established and maintained. Throughout both of the evaluation sessions he was engaging and friendly, he initiated spontaneous conversation frequently. It should be noted that Jon had been ill (i.e., earaches) prior to the first test session. After the first two-and-a-half subtests the examiner administered, Jon began to ask if we were almost done. Throughout both sessions he was restless, and moved around a lot and made disruptive noises. During both sessions, he requested restroom breaks in an effort to discontinue testing. When asked to manipulate test objects he typically banged the materials aggressively onto the table. During both testing sessions, Jon spoke aloud as he worked. For example, when looking at pictures, he would name or count them while pointing to them. When Jon was attentive, he focused and performed well; however, when his attention strayed, he generally gave up. When encountering a difficult item, he often noted, "It is too hard" or "I don't know." The results of this evaluation are considered to be a good estimate of Jon's current functioning level due to his good health and cooperation, that is, his behavior was typical of his classroom and home behavior. However, these results may not represent the best estimate of his overall intellectual potential due to considerable variability in his performance across measures.

Tests Administered

- Universal Nonverbal Intelligence Test (UNIT)
- Kaufman Assessment Battery for Children (K-ABC)
- Behavior Assessment System for Children (BASC)–Parent
- Conners' Rating Scales–Parent and Teacher Forms
- Children's Apperception Test (CAT)

Assessment Results and Clinical Impression

On the UNIT, Jon achieved a FSIQ of 97, and his overall intellectual functioning is ranked at the 42nd percentile for his age and is classified as Average. With 90% confidence, Jon's "true" FSIQ would be expected to be included in a range of scores between 91 to 103. (A true score is the hypothetical average that would be obtained upon repeated testing minus the effects of error, such as fatigue or practice.) Because Jon demonstrated considerable variability in the intellectual abilities assessed on the UNIT, his obtained FSIQ may not be the best representation of his overall intellectual abilities. In addition, Jon's performance on the UNIT may have been adversely affected by his recent illness, although he stated that he felt fine and experienced no pain at the time of testing. Jon's reasoning abilities (Reasoning Quotient = 118) are significantly better developed than his current memory skills (Memory Quotient = 79). Within the two scales (Memory and Reasoning) there was little subtest variability. This pattern of scale scores reflects a strength in reasoning, especially when Jon attends to visual aspects of a problem and when the elements of the problem are presented visually as a whole (i.e., part-whole relationship). He performed significantly less well when he was asked to solve problems by concentrating carefully and when he was asked to remember visually presented content.

On the K-ABC, Jon's Mental Processing Composite of 93 ± 6 is classified as Average. There is a significant difference between his Sequential Processing score, which is classified within the Average range, and his Simultaneous Processing score, which is within the low Average range of ability. Sequential processing tasks must be solved by arranging information in a sequential or serial order. Simultaneous tasks are spatial, analogic, or organizational in nature. Jon displayed a strength (Above Average) in quantitative short-term memory as measured on Number Recall, which is sequential. This task required him to repeat in sequence a series of numbers spoken by the examiner. This task requires short-term verbal memory, and suggests that his auditory short-term or working memory may be better developed than his visual short-term memory. In support of this finding, Jon earned a relatively low score on one of the K-ABC subtests that requires short-term visual memory. Jon also demonstrated a strength (Well Above Average) on Triangles, which is simultaneous. This task required him to combine several identical triangles into an abstract pattern to match a model. This performance is consistent with his Above Average UNIT performance on Analogic Reasoning and Cube Design subtests.

On the BASC Parent Rating Scale, completed by Jon's mother, one of the validity scores (F) was in the "Caution" range. The F index is a measure of the respondent's tendency to be excessively negative about the child's behaviors or self-perceptions and emotions. Jon's Externalizing Problems Composite, a measure of disruptive behavior, is rated significantly higher than his Internalizing Problems Composite, which is a measure of anxiety, depression, and similar emotional difficulties that are not marked by acting-out behavior. Jon's scores fall in the High range for Hyperactivity, Aggression, and Conduct Problems, as well as Depression. Jon's scores on the Adaptive Skills Composite are also in the High range. This composite consists of the Adaptability, Social Skills, and Leadership scales. On the Conners' Parent Rating Scale, also completed by Jon's mother, he was rated in the Very Much Above Average range on the Conduct Problem, Learning Problem, Impulsive-Hyperactive, and Hyperactivity Index. He was rated in the Slightly Below Average range on the Psychosomatic Index and Anxiety Index.

On the Conners' Teacher Rating Scale, completed by Jon's kindergarten teacher, he was rated in the Very Much Above Average range on the Conduct Problem, Emotional Overindulgent, and Hyperactivity Index. Jon was rated in the Much Above Average range on Hyperactivity; Above Average range on the Asocial Index; and Slightly Above Average range on Daydream-Attention Problem Index.

On the CAT, Animal Figures version, Jon's reference to the test characters on three out of ten pictures as "Tubby" and "Fatty" suggests a self depreciating self-image. On one picture he referred to a picture of a lion as the "Lion King," and he called himself the Lion King who did not feel good because animals were making fun of him, laughing, and saying bad words to him. The story "hero" had no friends and they called him "Stupid Head." On four pictures, Jon's explanations involved aggression, such as fighting, name calling, and biting. He told stories about fighting with his brother and about biting his brother's leg. On six pictures, Jon gave a one-or two- sentence explanation of what was on the picture and then quickly gave up by concluding "That's all!" In general, Jon's responses suggest themes of aggression, lack of friends, difficulty with impulse control, and negative self image. The short stories also demonstrate a short attention span and lack of task persistence.

Summary

Jon is 6 years 6 months old; he was referred because of home and school problems (e.g., inattention, aggression, failure to complete work). Jon's birth and developmental history are normal, but there is a history of ear infections and articulation difficulties. Overall, Jon's intelligence is classified within the Average range based on the K-ABC and the UNIT, though these test results may be an underestimate because of his high activity level, previous illness, and inattention. He demonstrated a strength in abstract thinking and analysis, and a weakness in memory, attention to detail, and concentration. He exhibited aggression and excessive activity during the evaluation. Jon's learning and behavioral problems may stem, in part, from his hearing problems. He requires considerable structure and works best when he is given novel, colorful material at his instructional level. Jon may work best if he is required to sit at the front of the class near the teacher. His teacher should provide clear visual cues and directions, and write things down whenever possible. Instructions may need to be repeated or clarified for him. Behavioral contracts based on task completion and non-aggressive physical behavior may be considered. Given the information obtained from observations in two settings, from behavior rating scales in both home and school settings, and from significant care givers, Jon qualifies for a diagnosis of Attention-Deficit/Hyperactivity Disorder, Combined Type (314.01), using criteria described in the *DSM-IV*.

Specific Recommendations

There are a number of recommendations that may be used to assist Jon at home and at school:

1. Provide visual cues when possible—write things down.
2. Have work structured in a step-by-step fashion.
3. Give clear, short directions, as well as short tasks.
4. Instructions may need to be repeated or clarified for him.
5. Develop a behavioral contract, with contingencies based on nonaggressive physical behavior and task completion.
6. Give praise for effort as well as completion of tasks.
7. Allow him frequent opportunities to be physically active within a

specified manner. For example, regular exercise breaks or carrying things for the teacher may help.

8. Give him a seat close to the front of the classroom.
9. Involve him in group activities under supervision and with good peer models.
10. Give him independent responsibilities.

It is recommended that his progress be monitored as the academic work becomes more time- and attention-consuming. It is also recommended that Jon has regular physical and audiological examinations. His pediatrician may consider medication for hyperactivity. Jon should be referred to a speech therapist for evaluation.

Attachment (Test Scores)
Test: UNIT   Date: 4/13/98

Subtests	Score
Symbolic Memory	5
Cube Design	13
Spatial Memory	9
Analogic Reasoning	13
Object Memory	6
Mazes	12

	Standard Score	Percentile	Descriptive Classification
Memory Quotient	79	8	Delayed
Reasoning Quotient	118	88	High Average
Symbolic Quotient	87	19	Low Average
Nonsymbolic Quotient	109	73	Average
Full Scale IQ	97	42	Average

Test: K-ABC   Date: 4/28/98

Global Scale	Standard Scores
Sequential Processing	102
Simultaneous Processing	90
Mental Processing Composite	93

Mental Processing Scaled Scores

Sequential Processing		Simultaneous Processing	
Hand Movements	8	Gestalt Closure	7
Number Recall	12	Triangles	14
Word Order	11	Matrix Analogies	7
		Spatial Memory	7
		Photo Series	8

Test: *BASC Parent Rating*   Date: 3/4/98

	T Score	90% Confidence Interval	Percentile Rank
Externalizing Problems			
Composite	87	82–92	99
Hyperactivity	74	66–82	98
Aggression	87	80–94	99
Conduct Problems	85	77–93	99

(continued)

Attachment (Test Scores) (*continued*)

	T Score	90% Confidence Interval	Percentile Rank
Internalizing Problems			
Composite	71	65–77	97
Anxiety	53	45–61	63
Depression	87	80–94	99
Somatization	58	49–67	82
Behavioral Symptoms			
Index	77	72–82	99
Atypicality	57	46–68	78
Withdrawal	55	46–64	74
Attention Problems	56	49–63	72
Adaptive Skills			
Composite	28	23–33	2
Adaptability	25	16–34	1
Social Skills	30	25–35	2
Leadership	38	32–44	13

Test: *Conners' Parent Rating*   Date: *4/28/98*

	T Score
A. Conduct Problem	97
B. Learning Problem	80
C. Psychosomatic	44
D. Impulsive-Hyperactive	80
E. Anxiety	40
F. Hyperactivity Index	89

Test: *Conners' Teacher Rating*   **Date: *4/28/98***

Scales	T Score
A. Hyperactivity	67
B. Conduct Problem	72
C. Emotional-Indul.	73
D. Anxious-Passive	45
E. Asocial	61
F. Daydream-Attention	60
I. Hyperactivity Index	73

Melissa Rifkin, Ph.D.
Psychologist

SUMMARY

Chapter 4 focused on describing: (a) the strengths and weaknesses of the UNIT; (b) clinical applications for several unique populations; and (c) the results of a case. This information is designed to help examinees hone their theoretical, empirical, and practical knowledge as they prepare to use the UNIT. Users will find the UNIT easy to administer, score, and interpret. The *Manual* includes a wealth of data describing the technical properties of the test and particularly fairness characteristics. In general, item and subtest properties are excellent, with few limitations. One salient limitation is the poor floor in the Abbreviated Battery for young cognitively limited children. The Riverside Publishing Company and the authors have developed a number of related materials, such as an administration video, a university training guide, and a training CD; scoring and interpretative software will be available in 2001.

☜ TEST YOURSELF ☞

1. **The age range for the UNIT standardization is**
   (a) 4 years to 16 years, 11 months
   (b) 5 years to 16 years, 11 months
   (c) 5 years to 17 years, 11 months
   (d) 6 years to 17 years, 11 months

2. **Which subtest yields a g loading less than .70?**
   (a) Mazes
   (b) Spatial Memory
   (c) Cube Design
   (d) Object Memory

3. **Which two subtests comprise the Abbreviated Battery?**
   (a) Cube Design and Spatial Memory
   (b) Cube Design and Object Memory
   (c) Cube Design and Symbolic Memory
   (d) Symbolic Memory and Matrix Analogies

4. **The two subtests with the poorest floors are**
   (a) Spatial Memory and Cube Design
   (b) Symbolic Memory and Cube Design
   (c) Spatial Memory and Matrix Analogies
   (d) Symbolic Memory and Matrix Analogies

5. **When compared with matched controls, a combined ESL and bilingual group earned higher mean _____ than _____ difference scores**
   (a) SQ : NSQ
   (b) NSQ : SQ
   (c) FSIQ : SQ
   (d) MQ : SQ

6. **In the case study, Jon's behavior resulted in a diagnosis of**
   (a) Learning Disability
   (b) Bipolar Disorder
   (c) Pervasive Developmental Disorder
   (d) Attention Deficit Hyperactivity Disorder

7. In the "Strengths and Weaknesses of UNIT Reliability and Validity" section it was indicated that _____ reliabilities are higher than _____ reliabilities

   (a) Split-half: test-retest
   (b) Test-retest: split-half
   (c) Predictive: test-retest
   (d) Predictive: split-half

8. Which of the following was listed as a developmental weakness?

   (a) Drawings are too colorful, hence distracting for young children
   (b) Drawings may not be engaging enough for young children
   (c) Development was not guided by stated goals
   (d) Development did not consider fairness issues

9. Development of the UNIT incorporated all of the following except

   (a) Bias panels
   (b) Use of statistical item analysis techniques to reduce bias in item selection
   (c) Use of confirmatory factor analyses to explore adherence to theoretical model
   (d) Use of path analysis procedures to determine adherence to theoretical model

10. Scoring on _____ subtest(s) allow(s) bonus points for speed

    (a) One
    (b) Two
    (c) Three
    (d) Four

Answers: 1. c; 2. a; 3. c; 4. b; 5. a; 6. d; 7. a; 8. b; 9. d; 10. b

Five

MULTIDIMENSIONAL NONVERBAL INTELLIGENCE TESTS: ADMINISTRATION, SCORING, AND INTERPRETATION OF THE LEITER-R

Of the various "nonverbal tests" there are two basic types. Those designed to assess a narrow conceptualization of intelligence, often using a matrices format, are referred to as unidimensional tests. Those designed to assess a broad conceptualization of intelligence, use a variety of administration formats, and tap multiple facets of children's intelligence are referred to as multidimensional. As described in Chapter 2, there are a plethora of unidimensional tests available; on the other hand, as mentioned in Chapter 3, there are only two comprehensive nonverbal tests of intelligence available, the UNIT and the Leiter-R. Chapter 5 provides a brief history of the Leiter-R, followed by descriptions of the theoretical model, the administration procedures, scoring criteria, and interpretation guidelines. The strengths and weaknesses of the Leiter-R are described in Chapter 6.

HISTORY AND DEVELOPMENT OF THE LEITER INTERNATIONAL PERFORMANCE SCALE–REVISED

The first published forerunner of the Leiter International Performance Scale appeared in 1929 (Roid & Miller, 1997), and five modifications of the scale were completed between 1930 and 1948. The 1948 Edition was published by Stoelting Company, and was the last revision actually undertaken by Dr. Russell G. Leiter. This version used wooden frames and stimulus blocks; the blocks were arranged by examinees to match or complete geometric patterns or symbols according to a rule the examinee was expected to discern. The latest version, completed under the guidance of Roid and Miller at the Stoelting Company, uses response easels and stimulus cards, but retains to a significant degree the "completion" format. Wooden frames have been replaced by three plastic frames molded into response easels; the original wooden blocks have been replaced by cards which can be placed into "slots" in the frames. Using these materials the original nature of the Leiter was retained, but important changes and modernizations were included (Roid & Miller, 1997).

According to the authors of the Leiter-R, it was designed to provide a culture-fair, nonverbal measure of intelligence, as was the original Leiter Performance Scale (Leiter, 1979). Roid and Miller (1997) define intelligence as measured on the Leiter-R as "the general ability to perform complex nonverbal mental manipulations related to conceptualization, inductive reasoning, and visualization" (p. 103). Included are tasks that assess spatial perception, nonverbal problem solving, attention to visual detail, classification of visual stimuli, and relationships among stimuli. The organizational scheme of the Leiter-R relies on 20 subtests forming two batteries; 10 subtests form the Visualization and Reasoning (VR) Battery and 10 the Attention and Memory (AM) Battery. In addition, there are four optional Social-Emotional rating scales: an Examiner Rating Scale, a Parent Rating Scale, a Self Rating Scale, and a Teacher Rating Scale. These address attention, activity level, organization/impulse control, sociability, sensory reactivity, emotions, anxiety, and mood, but are not part of the formal hierarchical organization of the Leiter-R. These scales provide social-emotional information and assess dimensions the authors refer to as "important adjuncts" to cognitive assessment (Roid & Miller, 1997).

The overarching model for the Leiter-R relies on the work of Carroll (1993), Horn and Cattell (1966), Gustaffson (1984), and Woodcock (1990), and assumes a hierarchical design with *g,* or general intelligence, at the apex. At the second level are broad factors such as Fluid Reasoning, Fundamental Visualization, Attention, and Memory. The Memory factor differentiates/converges at different ages, in part because subtests are introduced or removed from the battery as a function of age. Subtests are included at the third level and are assumed to assess even more unique components of the level two factors. The hierarchical model, as depicted in the *Leiter-R Manual* and in the *Stoelting Brief Nonverbal Intelligence Test Manual* (Roid & Miller, 1999) is shown in Rapid References 5.1 through 5.3. As is apparent from scrutiny of these figures, the factor-based models change slightly with age. According to the Leiter-R authors, there are three major factors at ages 2 through 5, including Fluid Reasoning,

≡≡ *Rapid Reference 5.1*

Leiter-R Model for Ages 2 to 5 Years

g

Fluid Reasoning	Fundamental Visualization	Attention
Repeated Patterns	Matching	Attention Sustained
Sequential Order	Picture Context	Associated Pairs
Classification	Figure Ground	Forward Memory
	Form Completion	

≡≡ *Rapid Reference 5.2*

Leiter-R Model for Ages 6 to 10 Years

g

Fluid Reasoning	Visual-Spatial	Attention	Associative Memory	Recognition Memory	Memory Span
RP	M	AS	AP	IR	FM
SO	FG	AD	DP	DR	RM
	FC				SM
	PF				VC
	DA				

Note. RP = Repeated Patterns; SO = Sequential Order; M = Matching; FG = Figure Ground; FC = Figure Completion; PF = Paper Folding; DA = Design Analogies; AS = Attention Sustained; AD = Attention Divided; AP = Associated Pairs; DP = Delayed Pairs; IR = Immediate Recognition; DR = Delayed Recognition; FM = Forward Memory; RM = Reverse Memory; SM = Spatial Memory; VC = Visual Coding. From Roid and Miller, 1997.

≡ *Rapid Reference 5.3*

Leiter-R Model for 11 to 20 Years

g

Fluid Reasoning	Visualization	Attention	Memory	Memory Span	Basic Visualization
RP	PF	AS	AP	FM	DA
SO	FR	AD	DP	RM	FG
FG				SM	FC
FC				VC	

Note. RP = Repeated Patterns; SO = Sequential Order; M = Matching; FG = Figure Ground; FC = Figure Completion; PF = Paper Folding; DA = Design Analogies; AS = Attention Sustained; AD = Attention Divided; AP = Associated Pairs; DP = Delayed Pairs; IR = Immediate Recognition; DR = Delayed Recognition; FM = Forward Memory; RM = Reverse Memory; SM = Spatial Memory; VC = Visual Coding. From Roid and Miller, 1997.

Fundamental Visualization, and Attention. At ages 4 to 5 a separate factor of Recognition Memory appears due to the introduction of the Immediate Recognition subtest. For examinees 6 to 10 years of age, the number of factors expands to six as the number of subtests increases. The factors are Reasoning, Visual/Spatial, Attention, Memory, Recognition Memory, and Memory Span. According to the *Leiter-R Manual*, for ages 11 to 20 there are five factors; however, according to D. Madsen of Stoelting (personal communication, March 30, 2000), the *Stoelting Brief Nonverbal Intelligence Test (SBIT) Manual* shows six factors, as depicted in Rapid Reference 5.3.

Goals for Leiter-R Development

Roid and Miller (1997) list four primary rationales for Leiter-R development, including: the need for early identification of cognitive delays, the need for measurement of small increments of cognitive improvement, the need for a reliable and valid measure of intelligence regardless of language or motor ability, and the need for information useful for transition planning for entering the

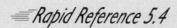

Rapid Reference 5.4

Goals for Leiter-R Development

1. Need to develop an instrument for early assessment of cognitive delays
2. Need to develop an instrument sensitive to small increments of cognitive improvement
3. Need to develop a reliable and valid instrument for use regardless of language and motor ability of examinee
4. Need to develop an instrument that could yield transition planning information for entering the work force

work force. All the goals focus on the need to provide cognitive assessment for examinees who cannot use the language. In fact, according to the *Leiter-R Manual,* nonverbal assessment should not require proficiency in perceiving, manipulating, and reasoning with words or numbers, printed materials, or any other material traditionally identified as verbal. Rather, assessment should rely on pictures, figural illustrations, and coded symbols, with administration instructions adapted via gestures and/or pantomime. See Rapid Reference 5.4 for a brief description of the Leiter-R goals.

Description of the Leiter-R

The Leiter-R provides 20 subtests and four rating scales, and allows various normalized standard scores. The subtests and rating scales produce raw scores, all of which can be translated to normalized scaled scores with a mean set to 10 and a standard deviation set to 3. Two IQ scores are available. One can be obtained from administration of a Brief IQ Screener consisting of four subtests; the second is referred to as a Full Scale IQ (FSIQ) and can be obtained from administration of six subtests. These subtests vary depending on age. The IQ scores can be calculated by summing subtest scores and converting these summed values to normalized deviation IQ standard scores, which use a mean set to 100 and a standard deviation set to 15.

Composite scores are also available for the rating scales. Raw scores from the rating scales are obtained using either a three or four choice Likert-rating format. Rating scales provide subscale scores in scale score units, ranging from 1 to 10, with 10 indicating average performance or "no clinical concern." Subscale raw scores (e.g., Attention, Activity Level, Sociability) are totaled to obtain *composites* for the ratings scales (Cognitive/Social and Emotions/Regulation), which are translated to normalized standard scores using the scores in the Conversion Tables in Appendix E of the *Leiter-R Manual*. Also, for each subtest and for the IQs Rasch-based ability estimates are available. These scores define abilities in a metric ranging from 380 to 560, with scores centered on beginning 5th grade (10 years, 4 months). The estimate of the degree of difficulty for each item can be expressed by its location on the growth curve, as shown in Appendix M in the *Leiter-R Manual*. Also, this index is sensitive to the rate at which the child is growing; scores can be compared from one administration to another. It is consistent across ages and across different collections of subtests. To obtain overall growth curve scores for subtests and Composite scores, use the tables in Appendixes N and M in the *Manual*.

For direct assessment, the Leiter-R provides a 20 subtest instrument, which is conveniently divided into two separate cognitive batteries, each with 10 subtests. The first battery, Visualization and Reasoning (VR), was designed for the assessment of examinees' fluid reasoning and visual-spatial abilities. The second battery, Attention and Memory (AM), was designed to assess examinees' attention, memory, and learning processes. The VR Battery produces five composites, which include a Brief IQ Screener (ages 2 to 20), an FSIQ (ages 2 to 20), Fundamental Visualization (ages 2 to 5), Fluid Reasoning (ages 2 to 20), and Spatial Visualization (ages 11 to 20). The AM Battery produces six composites, including a Memory Screener (ages 2 to 20), Recognition Memory (ages 2 to 10), Associative Memory (ages 6 to 20), Memory Span (ages 6 to 20), Attention (ages 6 to 20), and Memory Process (ages 6 to 20).

The two batteries and their respective composites produce standard scores with means of 100 and standard deviations set at 15. Leiter-R subtests produce scaled scores with means set at 10 and standard deviations of 3, with a range from 1 to 19. These scaled scores are obtained typically by summing the raw scores and taking the raw score sums to tables in the *Leiter-R Manual* in Appendix A (for the Visualization and Reasoning subtests), Appendix B (for the Attention and Memory subtests), or Appendix C1 (for the Attention and Memory Special Diagnostic scores) by age groups. Appendix D presents IQ equivalents for the sums of scaled scores for each of the IQ Scales. Scaled scores from the VR Battery Record Form can be used to organize all the subtests for summing of scores for the IQ or Composite scales. As with other multiple-subtest batteries, IQs and Composites are formed using the sum of scaled scores rather than the sum of raw scores. Finally, age equivalency scores are available by entering Appendix N with raw scores. However, the *Manual* suggests that this procedure is generally not recommended, as it only informs the examiner about the typical performance of the children in a specific age group who receive the same score as the child currently being evaluated. In addition, the age equivalence scores do not typically have equal-interval measurement properties and are therefore not useful for statistical manipulations.

VISUALIZATION AND REASONING SUBTESTS

1. *Figure Ground (FG)*. The Figure Ground subtest presents embedded figures on stimulus cards. The examinee is to identify the embedded figures within the more complex stimulus background presented on each stimulus plate. FG is appropriate for ages 2 to 21 years.

2. *Design Analogies (DA)*. Design Analogies presents abstract analogies in 2 × 2 and 2 × 4 matrix formats, as well as some matrices of more complexly designed formats. DA is appropriate for ages 6 to 21 years.

3. *Form Completion (FC)*. Form Completion is a puzzle solving type task that requires the examinee to assemble fragmented puzzle pieces to form a whole. FC is appropriate for ages 2 to 21 years.

4. *Matching (M)*. The Matching subtest requires examinees to discriminate and match visual stimuli that are presented on response cards with identical designs that are presented on a stimulus easel. M is appropriate for ages 2 to 10 years.

5. *Sequential Order (SO)*. The Sequential Order subtest presents pictorial or figural sequences, and the examinee is expected to identify from an array of options the designs that best complete the stimulus sequence. SO is appropriate for ages 2 to 21 years.

6. *Repeated Patterns (RP)*. The Repeated Patterns subtest presents pictorial or figural objects that are repeated in stimulus patterns; the examinee is required to use stimulus cards to complete each incomplete repeated pattern. RP is appropriate for ages 2 to 21 years.

7. *Picture Context (PC)*. The Picture Context subtest requires the examinee to identify the part of a picture that is missing within the

DON'T FORGET

Full Scale IQ, Brief IQ, Composites, and Subtest Scores available from the Leiter-R

Subtests for Brief IQ, Full Scale IQ, and Composites

Brief IQ	Full Scale IQ (Ages 2 to 5)	Full Scale IQ (Ages 6 to 20)
Figure Ground (FG)	Figure Ground (FG)	Figure Ground (FG)
Form Completion (FG)	Form Completion (FG)	Form Completion (FG)
Repeated Patterns (RP)	Repeated Patterns (RP)	Repeated Patterns (RP)
Sequential Order (SO)	Sequential Order (SO)	Sequential Order (SO)
	Matching (M)	Design Analogies (DA)
	Classification (C)	Paper Folding (PF)

Fluid Reasoning	Fundamental Visualization	Spatial Visualization
Sequential Order (SO)	Matching (M)	Design Analogies (DA)
Repeated Patterns (RP)	Picture Context (PC)	Paper Folding (PF)
		Figure Rotation (FR)

Memory Screening	Associative Memory	Memory Span
Associated Pairs (AP)	Associated Pairs (AP)	Forward Memory (FM)
Forward Memory (FM)	Delayed Pairs (DP)	Reverse Memory (RM)
		Spatial Memory (SM)

Attention	Memory Process	Recognition Memory
Attention Sustained (AS)	Forward Memory (FM)	Immediate Recognition (IR)
Attention Divided (AD)	Spatial Memory (SM)	Delayed Recognition (DR)
	Visual Coding (VC)	

Note. A description of the Leiter-R subtests by battery is given in this chapter.

context of the overall picture. PC is designed for examinees ages 2 to 5 years.

8. *Classification (C).* Classification is a subtest that requires the examinee to organize or classify materials according to their salient characteristics (e.g., shape, color, size). Classification is intended for ages 2 to 5 years.

9. *Paper Folding (PF).* Paper Folding requires the examinee to identify from several options what a paper figure would look like if it were folded. PF is a timed visualization subtest for examinees between 6 and 21 years old and requires the examiner to verbally "remind" the examinee of how much time remains to complete the task.

10. *Figure Rotation (FR).* The Figure Rotation subtest presents two- or three-dimensional objects, which the examinee must recognize after "mental rotation." FR is appropriate for examinees between the ages of 11 and 21 years.

ATTENTION AND MEMORY SUBTESTS

11. *Associated Pairs (AP).* One or more pairs of stimuli (e.g., colored shapes, single colored line drawings of objects) are presented for a 5- to 10-second exposure. After the brief exposure examinees are required to select the correct stimuli to complete each pair shown previously. AP is appropriate for children and adolescents ages 2 through 21 years.

12. *Immediate Recognition (IR).* In Immediate Recognition, a stimulus array depicting a variety of stimuli is presented for 5 seconds. After the brief exposure, the stimulus page is turned, revealing a second page with aspects of the first page absent. The examinee selects from response cards the stimuli that correctly match the initial stimulus arrangement. IR is appropriate for children between the ages of 4 and 10 years.

13. *Forward Memory (FM).* The examiner presents a number of stimuli to be recalled along with additional foils that are to be ignored. The examiner points to each relevant stimulus in a specified sequence, and encourages the examinee to replicate the sequence by pointing

to the stimuli in the same order as the examiner. FM is appropriate for ages 2 through 21 years.

14. *Attention Sustained (AS).* The Attention Sustained subtest requires the examinee to identify and cross out target stimuli embedded within rows of stimuli on a page that include both the target stimuli and several foils. AS is appropriate for ages 2 through 21 years.

15. *Reverse Memory (RM).* Using the same artwork as in FM, the examiner points to stimuli in a sequence. The examinee is required to point to the same stimuli in reverse order. RM is appropriate for ages 6 though 21 years.

16. *Visual Coding (VC).* Visual Coding presents pairs of stimuli within boxes arranged in an over and under design; that is, a target stimulus in the top row is paired with a second stimulus in the box below. Items are presented in rows with target stimuli in the top row, but the bottom row contains empty boxes. The examinee is to identify the proper stimulus that would appropriately be placed in each empty box to complete the stimulus pairs. VC is appropriate for ages 6 through 21 years.

17. *Spatial Memory (SM).* Spatial Memory presents a stimulus plate that depicts a variety of pictured objects within an increasingly complex grid. After a 10-second exposure the stimulus plate is removed from the examinee's view. The examinee is then directed to place response cards in the grid locations where each object originally had been presented. SM is appropriate for ages 6 through 21 years.

18. *Delayed Pairs (DP).* After an approximate 30 minute delay, the examinee's recall of objects depicted on the Associated Pairs subtest is assessed. Although AP is appropriate for the entire age range, the follow-up DP subtest is appropriate only for ages 6 through 21 years.

19. *Delayed Recognition (DR).* After an approximate 30 minute delay, the examinee's recall of objects depicted on the Immediate Recognition subtest is assessed. Like the IR subtest, DR is appropriate for ages 4 to 10 years.

20. *Attention Divided (AD).* In Attention Divided, a controlled number of objects are exposed to the examinee through "windows" on a movable insert that slides through a cardboard sheath. The

examinee points to the objects viewed in each trial exposure. Additionally, the examinee is taught a numerical card sorting activity, which is intended to compete with the card identification task for the examinee's attention. AD is appropriate for ages 6 through 21 years.

STANDARDIZATION AND PSYCHOMETRIC PROPERTIES OF THE LEITER-R

Standardization of the Leiter-R was conducted from two somewhat different normative samples for its two batteries, with only about one-third of the examinees administered both complete batteries. The VR Battery was normed on a total sample of 1,719 children, adolescents, and adults; the AM Battery normative sample included a smaller sample of 763 children, adolescents, and adults. All 763 examinees who were administered the AM Battery during the instrument's norming also were administered the entire VR Battery; these data provide the normative linkage between the two batteries.

Overall, the VR norms were based on an average sample size of slightly fewer than 100 individuals per age level (i.e., 19 age levels, 1,719 examinees). Importantly, fewer than 300 subjects *total* were included in the seven-year age span between 14 through 20 years, with an average of 41 subjects per age level. The AM Battery included fewer than 100 examinees at *every* age level across the entire age span, with samples that ranged from a low of 42 examinees at four age levels (i.e., 7, 8, 11, and 18 to 20 years) to a high of 86 children sampled at the 2-year-old age level. The Leiter-R authors justify these small sample sizes by claiming that the Leiter-R norm sample compares "favorably to that of a prominent memory and neuropsychological instrument, the *Wechsler Memory Scale–Revised* (Wechsler, 1987), which was standardized on a total sample of 316 subjects" (Roid & Miller, 1997, p. 143).

The Leiter-R normative sample was stratified on the basis of gender, race, socioeconomic status, community size, and geographic region, although the number and location of specific standardization sites were not reported in the *Leiter-R Examiner's Manual* (Roid & Miller, 1997). Representation of the standardization sample, as compared with the U.S. Census percentages, shows a fairly close match for the entire VR normative sample on each of the stratification variables (i.e., within 2% match); however, at individual age levels the samples are under- or overrepresented by as much as six to eight percent for individual stratification variables. For example, the authors indicate that 68.4% of the U.S. population is Caucasian, whereas only 60.2% of the ten-year-old sample is Caucasian (i.e., −8.2%); 73.9% of the 18- to 20-year-old sample is Caucasian (i.e., +5.5%). Across all the age levels, gender representation for the VR norms ranged from 46.7% male (ages 18 to 20 years) to 54.8% male at age 10. The AM sample, given its overall smaller size, has proportionately larger deviations from the U.S. population than does the larger VR sample. For example, the gender representation in the AM sample ranges from 39.6% male (ages 14 to 15 years) to 64.6% male at age 3, with disparity from the population parameters by approximately 11 to 15%. Over- and underrepresentation of the population on the remaining AM stratification variables also varies a bit more widely than for the VR sample across the age levels. For example, the examinee representation in the parent educational level, "Less than High School," ranges from 2.3% at age 6 to 26.7% at age 2; the national average is 19.8%. In general, the VR and AM samples match the U.S. population parameters fairly well at the total sample level; however, at individual age levels the disparities between the normative sample and the population are sometimes considerable.

Technical properties for the Leiter-R are generally good, with some variability. Average internal consistency (Coefficient Alpha) for the VR subtests across the age levels range from .75 to .90; average internal consistency for the AM subtests are generally lower and range from .67 to .87. Composite reliabilities for the Leiter-R VR Battery range from .88 to .93 (FSIQ .91 to .93); composite reliabilities for the AM Battery also tend to be lower than the VR composites and range from .75 to .93. Reliability estimates for the rating scales vary considerably depending on the particular scale. Average internal consistency estimates across the age levels range from .90 (Anxiety Section) to .97 (Attention Section) across the subscales of the Examiner Rating Scale; from .79 (Adaptation Section) to .90 (Sensitivity and Regulation Section) across the subscales of the Parent Rating Scale; from .91 (both the Temperament and Reactivity Sections) to .97 (Social Abilities Section) on the Teacher Rating Scale; and from .69 (Self-Esteem Section) to .77 (both the Organization/ Responsibility and Activity Level Sections) on the Self Rating Scale. See Rapid Reference 5.5 for a summary of average internal consistency coefficients for composites by ages.

≡ *Rapid Reference 5.5*

Average Internal Consistency Reliability Coefficients for Composites by Age

Leiter-R Composite	Ages 2 to 5	Ages 6 to 10	Ages 11 to 20
Brief IQ Screener	.88	.90	.89
Full Scale IQ	.92	.91	.93
Fundamental Visualization	.92	—	—
Fluid Reasoning	.88	.89	.89
Spatial Visualization	—	—	.91
Memory Screener	.87	.76	.75
Recognition Memory	.93	.87	—
Associative Memory	—	.81	.79
Memory Span	—	.88	.89
Attention	—	.79	.83
Memory Process	—	.86	.88

Note. From Roid and Miller, 1997.

Evidence for Leiter-R stability is presented in the *Examiner's Manual* for a sample of 163 children and adolescents (ages 2 to 20 years; median age 8 years, 11 months) for the VR Battery. The test-retest interval for the stability study was not identified. VR stability coefficients for the subtests across three broad age levels, as reported in the *Examiner's Manual,* range between .61 and .81 (ages 2 to 5); .70 and .83 (ages 6 to 10); and .65 and .90 (ages 11 to 20). VR composite stability coefficients range from .83 to .90 (ages 2 to 5); .83 to .91 (ages 6 to 10); and .86 and .96 (ages 11 to 20). It is important to note that these stability coefficients are possibly inflated due to significant expansion in the range of variability among examinees' test scores, and should be considered as favorable estimates. In this stability study, every subtest and scale produced standard deviations that were significantly greater than their respective normative standard deviations. For example, the standard deviation for the VR FSIQ was 30 at ages 11 to 20 years, which is twice the magnitude of the normative standard deviation of 15. It would have been helpful if both the corrected and obtained correlations had been reported in the Examiner's Manual.

In addition to the VR stability coefficients, the *Examiner's Manual* reports mean score differences for the VR Battery subtests and composites for the test-retest interval. Subtest gain scores vary considerably across the age levels and range from minor differences (e.g., .10 SD) to large, meaningful differences (e.g., 1.4 SD). The VR composites evidence similar gain scores that range from minor differences to gains of one-third to one-half standard deviation across the age levels. It is difficult to evaluate the stability of the VR Battery subtests' and composites' correlations and mean gain scores because the time interval between initial testing and post-testing is not reported in the *Examiner's Manual*.

An investigation of the stability of the AM Battery was also presented in the *Examiner's Manual,* and includes a sample of 45 children and adolescents (ages 6 to 17 years, median age 10 years, 11 months). As with the VR stability study, the AM study gives no indication of the test-retest interval. The AM Battery is generally less stable than the VR Battery, with corrected subtest coefficients that range from .55 to .85 (median = .615). AM composite stability coefficients range from .61 to .85 (median = .745). The practice effects on the AM subtests and composites also are generally larger than those found on the VR Battery and are typically about one-half standard deviation across the age span.

The *Leiter-R Examiner's Manual* reports eleven separate validity studies that describe the instrument's ability to discriminate among special groups (i.e., speech/language impaired; hearing impaired; traumatic brain injured; motor delayed; cognitive delayed; Attention Deficit Disordered; gifted; nonverbal learning disabled; verbal learning disabled; English as a second language, Spanish; and English as a second language, Asian or other). However, examination of the mean scores for these various groups suggests a possible problem with the sampling procedures. The mean FSIQs for the various 6- to 20-year-old samples are generally lower than anticipated (i.e., every sample except the gifted sample earned a mean FSIQ that was less than the test's normative mean of 100). Specifically, the gifted sample earned a mean FSIQ of 114.60, while all remaining special groups earned mean FSIQs of less than 90, except the two ESL groups. The preponderance of depressed group mean scores among special populations is inconsistent with the test's purported intention of fairly measuring cognitive impairment and delay.

A variety of concurrent validity studies also are reported in the *Leiter-R Examiner's Manual,* which include comparisons of the Leiter-R with other intelligence tests, such as the original Leiter, WISC-III, and selected subtests from the Stanford-Binet Intelligence Scale–Fourth Edition (Thorndike, Hagen, & Sattler, 1986). Although the correlation between the Leiter-R FSIQ and WISC-III FSIQ for a sample of normative, cognitively delayed, gifted, and ESL-Spanish cases is reported in the *Examiner's Manual* as .86, the standard deviations on both instruments employed in this study are between 23 and 26 IQ points. As with the Leiter-R stability studies, such an expanded range of variability would surely produce inflated validity coefficients between these two instruments. Also, similar to the stability study, the Leiter-R authors did not present both obtained and corrected correlations.

A number of small sample studies (i.e., 17 to 33 subjects) were conducted and reported in the *Leiter-R Examiner's Manual,* which compared the Leiter-R Brief IQ and FSIQ with aspects of various memory scales and achievement measures. The *Examiner's Manual* reports moderate to strong correlations (e.g., mostly .40s to .80s) between the Leiter-R Brief IQ and FSIQ, but the means and, most importantly, the standard deviations are not reported for these comparisons. Without means and standard deviations it is impossible to determine whether the tests produce comparable scores.

The authors suggest that the Leiter-R subtests fit the proposed underlying hierarchical *g* model that was used to design the instrument (p. 184). To the contrary, using Kaufman's (1979, 1994) criteria for "Good" (> .70), "Fair" (.50 to .69), and "Poor" (< .50) loadings on the *g*-factor, all of the Leiter-R subtests are classified as either Fair or Poor measures of *g,* except two. At ages 2 to 5 years, the Leiter-R *g* loadings range from .26 to .66, with a median of .595; *g* loadings range from .26 to .65 at ages 6 to 10 years (median = .45); and at ages 11 to 20 years, the *g* loadings range from .24 to .70, with a median of .56 (Roid & Miller, 1997, p. 192). The two subtests that qualify as Good *g*-loaders (i.e., Sequential Order and Paper Folding) meet Kaufman's criterion at one of the three broad age levels studied (i.e., ages 11 to 20 years); as with the remaining 18 subtests, these two latter subtests were classified as Fair or Poor measures of *g* at the remaining age levels.

Exploratory and confirmatory factor (LISREL and AMOS) analyses reported in the *Leiter-R Examiner's Manual* provide evidence for a reasonably good fit between a proposed four- or five-factor model. Given that the Leiter-R is founded on a two battery model, one might reasonably anticipate a two-factor fit instead. The model fit is fairly consistent across the age span, with support for a four-factor model at the younger age levels (i.e., ages 2 to 5 years) and a five-factor model from ages 6 through 20 years. The factors identified by the authors vary slightly in name and subtest composition across the age levels, but include such proposed abilities as Fluid Reasoning/Reasoning, Visualization/Visual Spatial, Attention, Recognition Memory, and Associative/Memory Span.

As part of a cross-battery approach to test interpretation, McGrew and Flanagan (1998) examined the prominence of cultural content embedded in various intelligence tests. McGrew and Flanagan classified eight of the 20 Leiter-R subtests as containing high levels of cultural content (e.g., pictures of culture-specific objects) and three more subtests were designated as having moderate levels of cultural content. As a result of the high degree of cultural content, these subtests may be of limited utility when used with children from non-U.S. or non-Western cultures.

HOW TO ADMINISTER AND SCORE THE LEITER-R

According to the *Leiter-R Manual,* users should adhere to the ethical standards published by their professional organizations (e.g., the American Psychological Association, Council for Exceptional Children). In addition, the *Manual* suggests that examiners should either be experienced in the use of intelligence tests, with training in graduate or professional-level courses, or be responsible enough to recognize their limitations and restrict their practice accordingly.

The *Leiter-R Manual* provides some general background information regarding appropriate physical conditions for assessment. Examiners are admonished to use a quiet environment and to minimize distractions and maximize comfort. Examiners are informed that on most subtests the examiner is positioned directly across the testing table from the examinee, rather than across the corner of the table; however, a few tests require that the examiner move to the examinee's side of the table. The *Manual* mentions the need for building rapport and for conducting the assessment according to standard administration procedures. Instructions for administration are located on the back of stimulus plates. Subtests are to be administered in the order they appear in the *Examiner's Manual* and on the Record Form, except when varying the order might facilitate a child's performance. There are three item types, requiring either: (a) placement of a Response Card; (b) arrangement of Manipulative Response Shapes; or (c) pointing responses on the Easel Pictures. Most items require the movement of the Response Cards into "slots" on the easel tray "frame." The frame has been integrated into the base of each easel. According to the *Manual*, the primary method for communication is pantomime, consisting of a combination of hand and head movements, facial expressions, and demonstration. Examiners are encouraged to be creative and flexible during pantomime of initial subtests, and to "feel free to extrapolate your own ways of communicating nonverbally" (Roid & Miller, 1997, p. 21).

The Leiter-R is administered in an almost completely nonverbal manner. It should be noted, however, that at least three subtests require the examiner to verbally indicate how much time remains during the timing of the subtests, and another subtest suggests that it "may require brief verbal supplementation" (Roid & Miller, 1997, p. 60). In addition, the collection of pantomimed gestures that are used to demonstrate the various Leiter-R subtests is vast and sometimes vague. Rather than employing a small set of standard gestures throughout all 20 subtests, the Leiter-R employs many general *and* unique gestures for subtests. The use of unique gestures for many subtests limits the generalization that examinees or examiners can make when progressing from subtest to subtest. Moreover, in many instances the *Examiner's Manual* provides only general directions without specifying accompanying gestures, such as "encourage the child to imitate you," "indicate nonverbally that each pair goes together," "indicate that the child should point to red apples only," or "indicate nonverbally that the child should point to all orange speed limit 55 signs AND red road construction signs seen on picture plate."

When gestures are described, they are sometimes broad and confusing. For example, the directions to one Leiter-R subtest state that the examiner should: "Indicate that card is 'mentally rotated' by touching your head and eyes and nodding 'Yes.' To demonstrate that cards should not be turned, begin to physically rotate card with your hand. Lightly tap that hand, with the other. Shake your finger back and forth to indicated (sic) 'No' to turning the card" (Roid & Miller, 1997, p. 44).

The *Manual* provides other directions for pointing (e.g., back and forth between the Response Cards and easel), gently touching the examinee (e.g., on the temple to signal eye contact), and using facial expressions to elicit "questioning." For example, the *Manual* notes: "This can be done by establishing eye contact, gesturing toward the card . . . with an open hand and raising one's eyebrow while saying silently to yourself 'your move!' or 'What's the answer?' You may wish to practice in front of a mirror or with a colleague to verify that your facial expression communicates questioning" (Roid & Miller, 1997, p. 22).

The examinee is encouraged to use other nonverbal signals, such as moving the hands or index fingers together, to indicate that shapes are to be "joined together." Rotation may be communicated by simply rotating the hand. The examiner may indicate "no" by putting his/her hand over the top of the stimulus materials and shaking his/her head from side to side. According to the *Manual,* in cases of deafness or severe sensory or motor impairment, some brief verbal (sign language) instructions may be needed.

Teaching Items and Scoring

Each subtest includes a "teaching trial," as the first item. On the teaching trial items examiners are permitted up to three repeated trials to demonstrate or guide the examinee through the process; examiners are encouraged to be creative in communicating task demands. Examiners are informed that generally, only one trial is permitted on all items except the teaching items. An exception can be made if an outside distraction occurs. Also, spontaneous self-corrections are scored as correct. Materials needed for administration of each subtest are listed on the instruction page, including the Easel Book number, the number of picture plates and response cards, and the specific manipulatives. See Rapid Reference 5.6 for a summary of Leiter-R components. Instructions are provided on the back of the easel pages. Information found on the back of each page includes administration directions, ages for which this item is a starting point or teaching trial (if applicable), correct responses, special administration notes if needed, and recommended position of the easel. For most of the subtests, items are scored either 1 (pass) or 0 (fail). Importantly, on items requiring sequencing, partial completion of a sequence is credited for most subtests (see the Subtest-by-Subtest Rules of Administration section below).

≡Rapid Reference 5.6

List of Leiter-R Components

Visualization and Reasoning (VR) Battery

Manual
Easel Books 1 and 2
Box of VR Response Cards
Manipulative Response Shapes
VR Record Forms with Examiner's Rating Scale

Attention and Memory (AM) Battery

Easel Book 3
Box of AM Response Cards
Manipulative Response Shapes
AM Record Forms with Examiner's Rating Scale
Response Booklets for the Attention Sustained subtest (ages 2 to 3, 4 to 5, 6 to 20)
Scoring keys for Attention Sustained Subtest (set of 12)
Colored picture plates for the Attention Divided subtest
Response Grids for the Spatial Memory subtest

Materials used with both Batteries

Stopwatch
Social-Emotional Rating Scales (Parent, Self, Teacher)
Growth Score Profile Sheets

Starting, Timing, Pacing, and Stopping Rules

Starting points are determined by the examinee's age, using three age groupings. Group A includes examinees from 2 to 5, Group B includes examinees from 6 to 10, and Group C includes examinees from 11 to 20. The starting point for each age group is presented on the first easel page of each subtest. A basal level is established for examinees if they are able to complete successfully the teaching trial; if that item is completed spontaneously the examinee is given credit for the item. If the examinee requires help on the teaching trial no credit is given. If the examinee is unable to complete the item successfully even with guidance, she/he returns to the starting point for the next younger age. If the examinee is unable to complete the teaching trials at the starting point for the youngest age for a particular subtest, a score of "0" is assigned for that subtest. Most of the subtests are untimed, with three exceptions, all from the VR Battery—Design Analogies, Paper Folding, and Figure Rotation. In the AM Battery, timing of exposure of easel pages is required for assessing short-term memory (e.g., 10-second exposures). In addition, on the Delayed Pairs and Delayed Recognition subtests, examiners are required to wait 30 minutes between an initial and delayed administration of the subtest. The *Manual* describes the use of a *pacing rule* for children who are unable to solve the assigned tasks, who are making guesses at items that are far too difficult, who are totally distracted, or who are extremely frustrated. The rule is employed after a maximum of 3 minutes; the examiner may discontinue the subtest after 3 minutes during which the examinee does not respond correctly. Stop criteria are made available at the top of each subtest on the Record Form and on the first page of instructions, and are based on performance on cumulative items, not consecutive items.

Subtest-by-Subtest Rules of Administration

Leiter-R norms allow for administration of a four- or a six-subtest battery in order to obtain IQs. Additional subtests may be administered to obtain other Composite Scores, depending on the examiner's needs and the referral question. In the following pages directions are provided for the administration of each subtest. However, examiners should keep in mind that the directions summarized here do not contain all the detailed information needed to actually administer the subtests. Because the directions are extensive, with considerable variation from one subtest to the next, examiners should read carefully the directions printed in the *Leiter-R Manual* before attempting to administer the test. The directions presented here represent the basic information examiners need, but because of space limitations, not all the subtleties are detailed. The first 10 subtests come from the Visualization and Reasoning Battery; the second 10 from the Attention and Memory Battery.

Rapid Reference 5.7 summarizes the specific *Figure Ground (FG)* subtest directions. This subtest is described in the *Manual* as a basic visual interference task, compounded by distractions and enhancements. For the FG subtest, stimulus cards are placed, centered, in front of the examinee and approxi-

≡Rapid Reference 5.7

Summary of Figure Ground Administration Rules

Starting Points

Ages 2 to 5: Item 1; use 2 cards for teaching trial item

Ages 6 to 10: Item 3; use 3 cards for teaching trial item

Ages 11 to 21: Item 5; use 3 cards for teaching trial item

Stop Rule

Six cumulative failures

Reversal Rules

If the examinee fails the teaching trial item at a particular starting point even after guidance, return to the starting point for the preceding age group.

Materials

Easel Book 1: 10 plates, 31 cards

---

mately 6 inches from the table's edge, in alphabetical order from the examiner's left to right. The examinee is expected to point to the place in the picture presented on the Easel Book where figures depicted on cards are hidden. After each response, return the cards to their original order.

The *Design Analogies (DA)* subtest is a measure of matrix reasoning. Administration requires that stimulus cards be centered in front of the examinee and approximately 6 inches from the table's edge, in alphabetical order from the examiner's left to right. The examinee is expected to point to the card that belongs in the empty square on the easel or in the correct "slot" on the tray. For the teaching trial items return the cards to their original order. This subtest requires special item administration directions for items 7, 12, 15–17, and 18 because the nature of the items changes (e.g., multiple cards must be selected rather than one, bonus points are added for speeded performance). Rapid Reference 5.8 summarizes administration directions.

The *Form Completion (FC)* subtest requires organization of disarranged or fragmented pieces, and requires flexibility. Administration requires that the examiner place shapes or cards in front of the examinee, centered and approximately 6 inches from the table's edge. The examinee is expected to put the shapes

≡ Rapid Reference 5.8

Summary of Design Analogies Administration Rules

Starting Points
Ages 2 to 5: Not administered
Ages 6 to 10: Item 1; Use 2 cards for teaching trial item
Ages 11 to 21: Item 8; use 4 cards for teaching trial item

Stop Rule
Seven cumulative failures

Reversal Rules
If the examinee fails the teaching trial item at a particular starting point even after guidance, return to the starting point for the preceding age group.

Materials
Easel Book 1: 18 plates, 72 cards

together or point to the picture of the objects "put together." This subtest requires special item administration directions for use of teaching items and for item 8. The examiner is directed to use items 1, 2, and 3 as teaching items for the youngest age group; also, the examiner is directed to switch to Easel Book 2 for item FC 9. Rapid Reference 5.9 summarizes administration directions.

The *Matching (M)* subtest requires the ability to match basic visuo-perceptual stimuli, with no memory component. For administration, the examiner places shapes or cards in front of the examinee, approximately 6 inches from the table's edge, in alphabetical order, from the examiner's left to right. The examinee is expected to match the stimulus materials to the examiner's model or to place the cards in the correct slot on the tray. For the teaching trial, items are returned to a different random placement in front of the child. After each item is administered, the examiner is instructed to hold each shape up to the easel and indicate that each shape also matches the easel. Credit is awarded for correct matches only. This subtest requires special item administration directions for items 1, 2, and 4. All these items can be used to teach for the youngest age group. Rapid Reference 5.10 summarizes administration directions.

≡ *Rapid Reference 5.9*

Summary of Form Completion Administration Rules

Starting Points

Ages 2 to 5: Item 1 in Easel Book 1
Ages 6 to 10: Item 6 in Easel Book 1
Ages 11 to 21: Item 9 in Easel Book 2

Stop Rule

Six cumulative failures

Reversal Rules

If the examinee fails the teaching trial item at a particular starting point even after guidance, return to the starting point for the preceding age group.

Materials

Easel Book 1: Items 1–8, 10 medium squares (4 blue, 6 red), 8 plates, 13 cards

≡ *Rapid Reference 5.10*

Summary of Matching Administration Rules

Starting Points

Ages 2 to 5: Item 1
Ages 6 to 10: Item 5
Ages 11 to 21: Not Administered

Stop Rule

Five cumulative failures

Reversal Rules

If the examinee fails the teaching trial item at a particular starting point even after guidance, return to the starting point for the preceding age group.

Materials

Easel Book 2: 16 shapes, 12 plates, 27 cards

The *Sequential Order (SO)* subtest assesses nonverbal reasoning ability, with an emphasis on rule generation related to seriation. Administration requires that the examiner place stimulus cards/shapes directly in front of the examinee, centered on the table, and approximately 6 inches from the table's edge, in alphabetical order from the examiner's left to right. The examinee is expected to match the stimulus materials to the examiner's model or to place cards in the correct tray slot. The examiner is directed to emphasize the importance of correct order. After the teaching trial, materials are rearranged in a different random order. Also, after items using shapes, the examiner is instructed to hold the shape up to the easel and show that each shape also matches the easel stimulus. Credit is given only for correct placement of the shapes. This subtest requires special item administration directions for item 2; for this subtest item 2 is a teaching item. Rapid Reference 5.11 summarizes administration directions.

The *Repeated Patterns (RP)* subtest assesses the ability to combine deductive reasoning with conceptual sequencing, and relies on rule generation. Administration requires that stimulus cards/shapes be placed directly in front of the

≡ Rapid Reference 5.11

Summary of Sequential Order Administration Rules

Starting Points
Ages 2 to 5: Item 1
Ages 6 to 10: Item 3
Ages 11 to 21: Item 5

Stop Rule
Seven cumulative failures

Reversal Rules
If the examinee fails the teaching trial item at a particular starting point even after guidance, return to the starting point for the preceding age group.

Materials
Easel Book 2: 6 shapes, 13 plates, 53 cards

≡ *Rapid Reference 5.12*

Summary of Repeated Patterns Administration Rules

Starting Points
Ages 2 to 5: Item 1
Ages 6 to 21: Item 5

Stop Rule
Six cumulative failures

Reversal Rules
If the examinee fails to independently complete the teaching trial item at a particular starting point even after guidance, return to the starting point for the preceding age group.

Materials
Easel Book 2: 17 shapes, 12 plates, 34 cards

examinee, centered on the table, approximately 6 inches from the table's edge, in alphabetical order from the examiner's left to right. The examinee is expected to put the shapes in the correct order, or place cards in the correct tray slot, based on cues found on the easel. The examiner is directed to emphasize the importance of correct order. After the teaching trial, materials are rearranged on the table and the child is encouraged to complete the item with no help. This subtest requires special item administration directions for item 4; for this subtest item 4 is a teaching item and items 5, 6, 7, 8, 9, 10, 11, and 12 require differing numbers of "distractor cards." Rapid Reference 5.12 summarizes administration directions.

The *Picture Context (PC)* subtest requires that the examinee fill in a missing part and relies on a deductive visual completion process. Administration requires that stimulus cards be placed directly in front of the examinee, centered on the table, approximately 6 inches from the table's edge, in alphabetical order from the examiner's left to right. The examinee is expected to point to the card(s) that relates to the empty box(es) on the easel picture. After the teaching trial, return the cards to their original positions. This subtest requires special item administration directions for item 2; for this subtest item 2 is also a

☰ *Rapid Reference 5.13*

Summary of Picture Context Administration Rules

Starting Points

Ages 2 to 5: Item 1
Ages 6 to 21: Do not administer

Stop Rule

Six cumulative failures

Reversal Rules

Begin with item 1 for ages 2 to 5; this subtest is not administered to ages 6 to 21.

Materials

Easel Book 2: 8 plates, 25 cards

☰ *Rapid Reference 5.14*

Summary of Classification Administration Rules

Starting Points

Ages 2 to 5: Item 1
Ages 6 to 21: Not administered

Stop Rule

Five cumulative failures

Reversal Rules

If the examinee fails to independently complete the teaching items even after guidance, go on to the next subtest.

Materials

Easel Book 2: 25 shapes, 11 plates, 15 cards

teaching item. Rapid Reference 5.13 summarizes administration directions.

The *Classification (C)* subtest requires sorting, and relies on abstraction and concept formation. Administration requires that stimulus cards/shapes be placed directly in front of the examinee, centered on the table, approximately 6 inches from the table's edge, in alphabetical order from the examiner's left to right. The examinee is expected to point to the correct tray slot, or to place cards in the correct tray slot. Cards relate to illustrations on the easel. This subtest requires special item administration directions for items 2 and 3; for this subtest these are also teaching items. Rapid Reference 5.14 summarizes administration directions.

The *Paper Folding (PF)* subtest requires visual-spatial abilities combined with inductive and deductive reasoning. Administration requires that the stimulus cards be placed directly in front of the examinee, centered on the table, approximately 6 inches from the table's edge, in alphabetical order from the examiner's left to right. The examinee is expected to place a card in the correct tray slot or point to the correct slot, based on the fit between the card and the illustration on the easel. That is, one of the cards shows an object (e.g., circle, square) that, when folded, looks like the picture on the easel. After the teaching trial, materials are rearranged on the table in their original position. Certain items require special administration directions; for example, some items require more cards than others (e.g., one card for items 1, 5–7; two cards for items 2–4, 8–12). Also, items 10–12 are timed and bonus points are given. Rapid Reference 5.15 summarizes administration directions.

The *Figure Rotation (FR)* subtest requires mental rotation of a three-dimensional figure. Administration requires that the stimulus cards be placed directly in front of the examinee, centered on the table, approximately 6 inches from the table's edge, in alphabetical order from the examiner's left to right. The examinee is expected to put the card(s) in the correct tray slot or to point to the appropriate card(s), based on a rotation rule shown on an easel. After the teaching trial, the teaching card is returned to its original position on the

---

≡Rapid Reference 5.15

Summary of Paper Folding Administration Rules

Starting Points
Ages 2 to 5: Not Administered
Ages 6 to 10: Item 1
Ages 11 to 21: Item 3

Stop Rule
Six cumulative failures

Reversal Rules
If the examinee fails to independently complete the teaching trial item at a particular starting point even after guidance, return to the starting point for the preceding age group.

Materials
Easel Book 2: 12 plates, 20 cards

table to allow the child an opportunity to complete the item independently. This subtest requires special item administration directions for items 12–14; these items are timed and bonus points assigned. Rapid Reference 5.16 summarizes administration directions.

The next 10 subtests come from the Attention and Memory Battery. The *Associated Pairs (AP)* subtest requires paired associates learning and taps short-term retention. Administration requires that stimulus cards/shapes be placed directly in front of the examinee, centered on the table, approximately 6 inches from the

≡Rapid Reference 5.16

Summary of Figure Rotation Administration Rules

Starting Points
Ages 2 to 5: Not administered
Ages 6 to 21: Item 1

Stop Rule
Seven cumulative failures

Reversal Rules
Ages 6 to 21 begins with item 1.

Materials
Easel Book 2: 14 plates, 14 cards

table's edge, in alphabetical order from the examiner's left to right. Beginning with item 5, the examiner exposes the target pair for 5 seconds. The page is then turned to expose dotted boxes. The examinee is expected to pair shapes/cards in sets of two. The child is expected to use either the examiner's model or the stimuli pictured on the easel. After the teaching trial, materials are rearranged on the table in a different random order. This subtest requires special item administration directions for several items. For example, item 2 is also a teaching item. Beginning with item 5, the pair is exposed for 5 seconds only. For items 9–12 the stimulus page is shown for 10 seconds, and the examinee has a total of 20 seconds to respond. As indicated in the *Leiter-R Manual,* other minor adjustments are needed for these items. Rapid Reference 5.17 summarizes administration directions.

The *Immediate Recognition (IR)* subtest assesses the ability to form a rapid visual image and then recognize its elements after a short delay. Administration of each new item requires that the easel page be turned to Plate "a." Position the easel to indicate a new item is about to be administered. Expose Plate "a" for 5 seconds. Turn to Plate "b" and center cards in front of the child, approximately 6 inches from the table's edge, in alphabetical order from the examiner's left to right. The examinee is expected to independently select the

≡ Rapid Reference 5.17

Summary of Associated Pairs Administration Rules

Starting Points

Ages 2 to 5: Item 1
Ages 6 to 21: Item 5

Stop Rule

Ten cumulative failures

Reversal Rules

If the examinee fails to independently complete the teaching trial item at a particular starting point even after guidance, return to the starting point for the preceding age group.

Materials

Easel Book 3: 9 shapes, 12 plates, 52 cards

card(s) that represents the missing illustration(s). After the teaching trial, the examiner picks up the cards and flips back to Item 1a. Expose it for 5 seconds, then turn to Item 1b. Indicate that the child should independently demonstrate which of the three cards belongs on Item 1b. This subtest requires special item administration directions for Item 16; it is exposed for 10 seconds. Rapid Reference 5.18 summarizes administration directions.

The *Forward Memory (FM)* subtest assesses sequential memory and requires sustained attention and organization. Administration requires that the examiner center the easel in front of the examinee, approximately 6 inches from the table's edge. The examinee is then expected to point to a series of pictures on the easel in the same order as the examiner. This subtest requires special item administration directions for item 2; for this subtest item 2 is also a teaching item. Rapid Reference 5.19 summarizes administration directions.

The *Attention Sustained (AS)* subtest can be characterized as a cancellation task, and assesses visual prolonged attention using visual scanning and motoric inhibition. Administration requires centering the appropriate AS Booklet directly in front of the examinee, so that only one page is shown at a time. The examinee is expected to cross out during the allotted time as many target

≡Rapid Reference 5.18

Summary of Immediate Recognition Administration Rules

Starting Points

Ages 2 to 3: Not administered
Ages 4 to 10: Item 1
Ages 11 to 21: Not administered

Stop Rule

Eight cumulative failures

Reversal Rules

This subtest is administered to ages 4 to 10 only.

Materials

Easel Book 3: 32 plates, 57 cards

≡Rapid Reference 5.19

Summary of Forward Memory Administration Rules

Starting Points

Ages 2 to 5: Item 1
Ages 6 to 10: Item 3
Ages 11 to 21: Item 5

Stop Rule

Six cumulative failures

Reversal Rules

If the examinee fails to independently complete the teaching trial item at a particular starting point even after guidance, return to the starting point for the preceding age group.

Materials

Easel Book 3: 6 plates

≡Rapid Reference 5.20

Summary of Attention Sustained Administration Rules

Starting Points

Ages 2 to 3: Booklet A

Ages 4 to 5: Booklet B

Ages 6 to 21: Booklet C

Stop Rule

All the Booklet pages associated with a particular age should be administered to a child.

Reversal Rules

If the examinee cannot perform the teaching trial item at a particular starting point discontinue the subtest..

Materials

The appropriate booklet, stopwatch, and colored marker

---

pictures as possible that look like the picture presented at the top of the page. Specific timing instructions are printed at the top of each page. The examiner is admonished not to demonstrate crossing out on the actual test pages. Rapid Reference 5.20 summarizes administration directions.

The *Reverse Memory (RM)* subtest assesses working memory. The examiner is required to center the easel in front of the examinee and point to the pictures in the order shown in the Record Booklet. The examinee is expected to point to the pictures in the reverse order. Rapid Reference 5.21 summarizes administration directions.

The *Visual Coding (VC)* subtest taps persistence, sustained attention, working memory, and, to a lesser extent, reasoning. Administration requires that the examiner place stimulus cards directly in front of the examinee, centered on the table, approximately 6 inches from the table's edge, in alphabetical order from the examiner's left to right. The examinee is expected to put the cards in the correct tray slots, or indicate which card(s) belong(s) in the empty square on the easel, based on a key that appears on the easel. After the teaching trial,

≡ Rapid Reference 5.21

Summary of Reverse Memory Administration Rules

Starting Points
Ages 2 to 5: Not administered
Ages 6 to 21: Item 5

Stop Rule
Six cumulative failures

Reversal Rules
If the examinee fails to complete independently the teaching trial item at the starting point for ages 2 to 5, discontinue the subtest.

Materials
Easel Book 3: 3 plates

materials are rearranged into their original position. This subtest requires special item administration directions for items 2 and 9; for this subtest item 2 is also a teaching item. Item 9 allows the examiner to provide additional teaching clues because the nature of the task changes for items 9–13. Also, note that several items use distractor cards (items 4, 5, 6, 9, 10, 11, 12, and 13). Rapid Reference 5.22 summarizes administration directions.

The *Spatial Memory (SM)* subtest is sometimes considered a visual analog to the digit span subtest, and assesses immediate memory for spatial location. Administration requires centering a blank grid in front of the examinee, close to the easel book. Turn to Plate "a" and show it to the examinee for 10 seconds. Then turn to Plate "b." Place the appropriate cards between the examinee and the grid, in alphabetical order from the examiner's left to right (as he/she faces the examinee). The examinee is expected to place cards on the grid in the same location where they were illustrated on Plate "a." There are five grids used for this subtest; grid 1 is used for items 1 and 2, grid 2 is used for items 3–4; grid 3 for items 5–9; grid 4 for items 9–15 (sic); grid 5 for items 15–20 (sic). The examiner is directed to put cards into two rows when the num-

≡ Rapid Reference 5.22

Summary of Visual Coding Administration Rules

Starting Points

Ages 2 to 5: Not administered
Ages 6 to 10: Item 1
Ages 11 to 21: Item 5

Stop Rule

Six cumulative failures

Reversal Rules

If the examinee fails to independently complete the teaching trial item at a particular starting point even after guidance, return to the starting point for the preceding age group.

Materials

Easel Book 3: 13 plates, 62 cards

≡ Rapid Reference 5.23

Summary of Spatial Memory Administration Rules

Starting Points

Ages 2 to 5: Not administered
Ages 6 to 10: Item 1
Ages 11 to 21: Item 3

Stop Rule

Six cumulative failures

Reversal Rules

If the examinee fails to independently complete the teaching trial item at a particular starting point even after guidance, return to the starting point for the preceding age group.

Materials

Easel Book 3: 20 plates, 13 cards, 5 laminated blank grids

ber of cards is greater than six.. Rapid Reference 5.23 summarizes administration directions.

The *Delayed Pairs (DP)* subtest requires "long-term" retrieval of information stored for at least 30 minutes. It may also tap incidental learning to some extent. Administration is accomplished by placing stimulus cards directly in front of the examinee, centered on the table, approximately 6 inches from the table's edge, in alphabetical order from the examiner's left to right. The examinee is expected to put the shapes in the correct tray slot or indicate which cards belong in the empty squares on the easel. This subtest is designed to determine how much the examinee remembers from subtest 11 (Associated Pairs; AP). The examiner is directed to administer DP in the same testing session as AP, to require at least 30 minutes between the start of AP and DP, and to stop administering items at the "stop" point obtained on AP, even if 10 responses have not been failed. Also, only easel pages that require a response are shown to the examinee. As with the AP subtest, items 9–12 allow 20 seconds for a response. Rapid Reference 5.24 summarizes administration directions.

The *Delayed Recognition (DR)* subtest assesses long-term memory and incidental learning. Administration is accomplished by placing stimulus cards directly in front of the examinee, centered on the table, approximately 6 inches from the table's edge, in alphabetical order from the examiner's left to right. The examinee is expected to select cards that represent the missing illustration(s) on the easel. This subtest is designed to determine how much the examinee remembers from subtest 12 (Immediate Recognition; IR). The examiner is directed to administer DR in the same testing session as IR, to require at least 30 minutes

═Rapid Reference 5.24

Summary of Delayed Pairs Administration Rules

Starting Points
Ages 2 to 5: Not administered
Ages 6 to 21: Item 5

Stop Rule
Ten cumulative failures, but no further than the stop point on Associated Pairs

Reversal Rules
If the examinee fails to appreciate the concept of remembering the pairs, discontinue this test.

Materials
Easel Book 3: 12 plates, 46 cards

≡Rapid Reference 5.25

Summary of Delayed Recognition Administration Rules

Starting Points

Ages 2 to 3: Not administered

Ages 6 to 10: Item 1

Ages 11 to 21: Not administered

Stop Rule

Eight cumulative failures, but not beyond stop point for Immediate Recognition

Reversal Rules

If the examinee fails to appreciate the task demands discontinue this subtest.

Materials

Easel Book 3: 16 plates, 57 cards

between the start of IR and DR (unless Associated Pairs and Delayed Pairs have been administered, in which case no additional waiting time is required), and to administer only those items administered in IR. The stop point is eight cumulative failures and the examiner is directed to administer no new items (i.e., any not administered in IR). Also, only easel pages that require a response are shown to the examinee. Rapid Reference 5.25 summarizes administration directions.

The *Attention Divided (AD)* subtest assesses the ability to hold in active memory two or more ideas simultaneously. Administration is somewhat challenging, and requires that the examiner become extremely familiar with the content before attempting an evaluation. The examinee is required to perform two tasks (and obtains two scores on each item), alternating between them. The examinee sorts a deck of cards in numerical order and points to a frame through which the examiner pulls various pictures at a constant but fairly slow rate. The examiner is instructed to pause 4–5 seconds between pictures. The examiner can use short sentences to help explain the alternating nature of this subtest. The items are timed, and timing instructions are located in the Record Booklet. Rapid Reference 5.26 summarizes administration directions.

≡ Rapid Reference 5.26

Summary of Attention Divided Administration Rules

Starting Points
Ages 2 to 5: Not administered
Ages 6 to 21: Item 1

Stop Rule
The *Leiter-R Manual* instructs the examiner to discontinue if the examinee cannot understand the nature of the task after using the teaching trials.

Reversal Rules
If the examinee fails to appreciate the task demands, discontinue this test.

Materials
Easel Book 3: 3 picture plates (AD1, AD2, AD3), 7 picture cards, a set of sorting cards numbered 1–20, frame from the picture plates—the frame is mounted on the easel support

Test Booklets and *Manual*

There are two Record Forms, one for the Visualization and Reasoning Battery and one for the Attention and Memory Battery. In addition, there is a Growth Score and Rating Scales Profile on one record form. Test booklets include work space for converting raw scores to standard scores, spaces to record IQs, composites, percentiles, growth composites, standard error of measurement, confidence intervals, and profile figures to be used for composite scores and subtests.

In addition to providing the essential elements of administration and scoring, interpretation, and supportive statistical evidence, the *Examiner's Manual* provides general information about adapting the administration of the Leiter-R for exceptional populations, suggesting that "It may be necessary to create unusual methods by which the child can communicate their (sic) answers to test items" (p. 76). The authors recognize that test adaptation also affects the value of the norms, and caution that the Leiter-R norms may be "radically changed in the adaptation process." The value of adapting the Leiter-R is unclear, as are the conditions under which adaptation would be justifiable.

LEITER-R INTERPRETATION

According to the *Leiter-R Manual,* interpretation may occur at five levels in a hierarchical fashion. The strategies described in this section rely to some extent on the suggestions provided by Roid and Miller (1997), but are also drawn from some of the traditional interpretive strategies found in the intelligence testing literature (e.g., Bracken & McCallum, 1998; Kaufman, 1979; Kaufman & Lichtenberger, 1999). Using the hierarchical method advocated by Roid and Miller requires that the overall nonverbal IQ be interpreted first as a measure of g. Of course, this score should be couched within a band of error.

Next, Growth Scores may be interpreted as an index of intrapersonal growth and development over time, if desired. The examinee's performance is defined by tasks on the scales that are mastered (or not). The next level of interpretation uses Composite Scores to examine clusters of ability such as Memory and Visual/Spatial Abilities; according to the Leiter-R authors these scores may be used predictively (e.g., to predict attention problems or hyperactivity). The next level requires examination of subtest scores. Finally, it is possible to examine special Attention/Memory Battery Diagnostic Scores as well as scores from the Rating Scales for increasingly detailed accounts of performance. The interpretive strategies we describe follow the general hierarchical strategy as outlined by Roid and Miller, but focus extensively on interpretation of the IQs and Composite and Subtest Scores, and relatively less on the growth curve scores and rating scales.

There are nine cognitive composites available from the Leiter-R and two composites from each of the rating scales. The three composite scores on the VR Battery include one reasoning scale (Fluid Reasoning, consisting of RP + SO) and two visualization scales (Fundamental Visualization, consisting of M + PC, ages 2 to 5; Spatial Visualization, consisting of DA + PF + FR, ages 11 to 20). The six composite scores from the AM Battery include a Memory Screener (consisting of AP + FM, ages 2 to 20); three other memory scales (i.e, Recognition Memory, consisting of IR + DR, ages 4 to 10; Associative Memory, consisting of AP + DP; Memory Span, consisting of FM + RM + SM); one attentional scale (Attentional Composite, consisting of AS + AD); and one clinical cluster, which may be used to predict Attention-Deficit/Hyperactivity Disorder (ADHD) (the Memory Process Composite, consisting of FM + SM + VC). The rating scales include composites entitled Cognitive/

Social and Emotional/Regulation. The rating scales are designed to be sensitive to various characteristics of interest. See Rapid Reference 5.27 for a listing of the subtests included on each scale. The following section describes the specific steps for interpretation of Composite Scores from the Visualization and Reasoning and the Attention and Memory Batteries, using standard scores.

The Six Steps of Leiter-R Interpretation

Step 1: Interpret the Full Scale IQ and Composite Scores First The first stage of Leiter-R interpretation requires describing the examinee's performance at the composite level (i.e., FSIQ, Fundamental Visualization) by using standard scores, confidence intervals, percentile ranks, and, if needed, Normal Curve Equivalents. Quantitative descriptions are based on interpretation of obtained scores relative to population parameters, and by inference, relative to peers the examinee's age. For example, the Leiter-R composite standard scores are based on a population mean of 100 and a standard deviation of 15. Because intelligence is a construct that fairly well conforms to the traditional normal bell curve, standard scores on the Leiter-R scales can be compared to IQs and other standardized scores obtained on other tests based on the same metric (i.e., M = 100, SD = 15). IQs may be categorized qualitatively using the descriptive labels from the *Leiter-R Manual:* Severe Delay (30–39); Moderate Delay (40–54); Very Low and Mild Delay (55–69); Low (70–79); Below Average (80–89); Average (90–109); Above Average (110–119); High (120–129); Very High/Gifted (130–170).

Variability in obtained scores comes from two sources—reliable variance and error variance—and the error associated with the composite scores should be considered and communicated to clarify the difference between the examinee's obtained scores and his or her "hypothetical true scores." Obtained scores should be considered within a band of error that frames the obtained score. This band of error, referred to as the standard error(s) of measurement (SEm), shifts depending on the level of confidence desired (e.g., 68%, 95%, 99%). Confidence intervals built around obtained scores define the probability that a given range of scores would include the examinee's "true" score. A true score is defined as the hypothetical average that would be obtained upon repeated testing, minus the effects of error, such as practice or fatigue. For the Leiter-R, the band of error (SEm) can be found in Figures

Subtests Included on the Four Leiter-R Rating Scales

Examiner Scale	Parent Scale	Self Rating Scale	Teacher Scale
Attention	Attention	Organization	Attention
Organization/Impulse Control	Activity Level	Activity Level and Moods	Organization/Impulsivity
Activity Level	Impulsivity	Feelings and Reactions	Activity Level
Sociability	Adaptation	Self Esteem	Social Abilities
Energy and Feelings	Mood and Confidence		Mood and Regulation
Mood and Regulation	Energy and Feelings		Temperament
Anxiety	Social Abilities		Reactivity
Sensory Reactivity	Sensitivity and Regulation		Adaptation

9.14–9.17 in the *Leiter-R Manual*. For subtests, the SEm approximates 1.0; for the VR Battery the values across all ages for the various Composite Scores and IQs are 5 (IQ Screen), 4 (FSIQ), 5 (Spatial Visualization), 5 (Fluid Reasoning), and 4 (Fundamental Visualization). For the AM Battery the standard errors of measurement round to 5 (Recognition Memory), 7 (Associative Memory), 5 (Memory Span), 5 (Memory Process), 7 (Attention), and 7 (Memory Screen). Values are reported to two decimal places and by age in the Figures in the *Leiter-R Manual*, but the rounded values reported here are sufficient for most purposes.

Step 2: Determine the Statistical Significance of Composite Score Differences The Leiter-R contains two primary batteries: Visualization and Reasoning (VR), and Attention and Memory (AM). According to the interpretation strategies described in the *Leiter-R Manual*, the batteries are interpreted independently for the most part. That is, composite scores and subtests may be compared and contrasted within the two batteries, but comparisons across the batteries are very limited. Appendix F3.1 in the *Leiter-R Manual* reports only four comparisons: Brief IQ and Memory Screener, Brief IQ and Memory Process, FSIQ and Memory Screener, and FSIQ and Memory Process. Rapid Reference 5.28 shows the relevant values from that Appendix, by age. Of course, because the

≡Rapid Reference 5.28

Differences between VR and AM IQ/Composite Scores Required for Statistical Significance at the .05 Level by Age Group

Ages	Brief IQ Screener vs. Memory Screener	Full Scale IQ vs. Memory Screener	Brief IQ Screener vs. Memory Process	Full Scale IQ vs. Memory Process
2 to 5	14.70	13.47	—	—
6 to 10	17.14	16.89	14.40	14.10
11 to 20	17.64	16.63	14.10	12.81

Note. From Roid and Miller, 1997.

psychometric scales use the same metrics across the two batteries (mean set to 100, standard deviation to 15), it may be possible to make other comparisons, as would be possible between any two tests using the same metric properties.

Most users of the Leiter-R will be interested in obtaining an IQ and may only administer the VR Battery. Because the FSIQ includes aspects of reasoning, visualization, and spatial abilities, and is typically the best representation of the examinee's overall or global intelligence, it is the first score to be examined. In fact, many users interested primarily in obtaining an IQ, will administer only those six subtests necessary to obtain that score. However, whenever there is significant variability in an examinee's subtest and/or scale scores, the FSIQ may not serve as a good representation of global ability. To determine the representativeness of the FSIQ as an estimate of overall intellectual ability, the examiner should first consider the variability of the Leiter-R global or composite scores within the FSIQ Scale (e.g., Fluid Reasoning versus Spatial Visualization). If these composite or scale scores show considerable variability (i.e., significant difference among themselves), these differences should be interpreted *if* they are also abnormally large (see Step 3), and the FSIQ should not be considered a good estimate of overall functioning.

How large should differences between composite or scale scores be before the differences are considered important? If the difference between two composites or scales is statistically significant, that is, so large that it would not likely occur by chance alone, such a difference should be considered important, at least initially. After Kaufman and Lichtenberger (1999), we recommend that a probability level of .05 be used to determine significance; some examiners may choose a more conservative criterion (e.g., .01). The *Leiter-R Manual* recommends (and reports) only the .05 level, and we follow suit. However, statistically significant differences are not necessarily clinically meaningful nor rare. If differences exist, they should be checked to determine how rare they are in the population, as in Step 3. See Rapid References 5.29 and 5.30 for the VR and AM Batteries for values considered significant at the .05 level and Rapid References 5.31 and 5.32 to determine "rareness." (The logic described in Steps 1 through 6 may be applied to both batteries, and information necessary to interpret composites and subtests within both batteries is provided. Remember, however, that the AM Battery does not provide a single primary score analogous to the FSIQ.)

Step 3: Determine whether the Differences between Composite Scores are Abnormally Large
The relative frequency with which significant score differences occur within

≡ *Rapid Reference 5.29*

IQ and VR Composite Score Differences Required for Statistical Significance at the .05 Level by Age Group

Age	Brief IQ Screener vs. Spatial Visualization	Brief IQ Screener vs. Fluid Reasoning	Brief IQ Screener vs. Fundamental Visualization	Full IQ Scale vs. Spatial Visualization	Full IQ Scale vs. Fluid Reasoning
2 to 5	—	14.40	13.15	—	13.15
6 to 10	—	13.47	—	—	13.15
11 to 20	13.15	13.79	—	11.76	12.47
All	—	13.79	—	—	12.81

Age	Full IQ Scale vs. Fundamental Visualization	Spatial Visualization vs. Fluid Reasoning	Fluid Reasoning vs. Fundamental Visualization
2 to 5	11.76	—	13.15
6 to 10	—	—	—
11 to 20	—	13.15	—
All	—	—	—

Note. The IQ and VR Composite Scales are: Brief IQ Screener (FG + FC + RP + SO); Full Scale (six Subtests); Fluid Reasoning Composite (RP + SO); Fundamental Visualization (M + PC); and Spatial Visualization Composite (DA + PF + FR). From Roid and Miller, 1997.

Data and Table Copyright © 1997 by Stoelting Co. All rights reserved. Used with permission.

the population is another important indicator of variability. Relative frequency of differences addresses a separate issue from statistical significance. As mentioned above, statistical significance is described as the probability that the obtained score difference would be expected to occur in the population by chance alone. However, differences of that magnitude may occur in the normative population with considerable frequency due to real differences in

≋ Rapid Reference 5.30

AM Composite Score Differences Required for Statistical Significance at the .05 Level by Age Group

Age	Recognition Memory vs. Memory Screener	Associative Memory vs. Memory Span	Associative Memory vs. Memory Process	Associative Memory vs. Attention	Associative Memory vs. Memory Screener	Memory Span vs. Memory Process
2 to 5	13.15	—	—	—	—	—
6 to 10	17.88	16.37	16.89	18.59	19.28	14.99
11 to 20	—	16.63	16.89	18.12	19.94	14.10
All	16.10	16.37	16.89	18.36	18.59	14.40

Age	Memory Span vs. Attention	Memory Span vs. Memory Screener	Memory Process vs. Attention	Memory Process vs. Memory Screener	Attention vs. Memory Screener
2 to 5	—	—	—	—	—
6 to 10	16.89	17.64	17.39	18.12	19.72
11 to 20	15.56	17.64	15.83	17.88	19.05
All	16.10	16.37	16.63	16.89	18.36

Note. The AM Composite Scales are: Recognition Memory (IR + DR); Memory Screener (FM + AP); Associative Memory (AP + DP); Memory Span (FM + RM + SM); Memory Process (FM + SM + VC); and Attention (AS + AD cards). From Roid and Miller, 1997.

the abilities of individuals within the population, rather than to chance factors. Also, differences occur in both directions. Examiners should check Rapid Reference 5.31 and 5.32 to find the relative frequency of score differences in the population for differences ranging from 5 to 25 for the AM and VR Batteries. We recommend that point differences be considered "abnormally large" if they occur only in the most extreme 15% of the population (after Naglieri & Kaufman, 1983). If there is one or more abnormally large difference among the scale scores (e.g., Fluid Reasoning is significantly higher than Spatial Visualization), the resulting Leiter-R FSIQ is a less than optimal index of the examinee's overall abilities. In that case, scales should be interpreted as important indicators of (independent) abilities in their own right. (Rapid References 5.31 and 5.32 show cumulative percentages of the VM and VR Batteries for extreme Composite Score differences.) There is one caveat, however. If there is abnormal scatter among the subtests within a particular global scale, that scale should not be interpreted as a unique and cohesive entity. Scatter is indicated by subtracting the lowest subtest score from the highest within the global area. If this range of scores is equal to or greater than nine points, the scatter may be considered abnormally large, that is, so large that only approximately 15% of the standardization sample earned a value this large or larger.

Step 4. Interpret the Significant Strengths and Weaknesses of the Profile   Step 4 begins the actual examination of the theoretical underpinnings of the test. That is, if the global scales or composites exhibit statistically significant and abnormally large difference, interpretation proceeds along theoretical lines (e.g., Fluid Reasoning greater than Spatial Visualization or Associative Memory greater than Attention). Examinees who exhibit particular patterns of performance would be expected to achieve differentially. Also, non-Leiter-R based models may be important to consider, and that possibility is investigated empirically in Step 5. For example, application of the Simultaneous-Successive model of processing, the Cattell-Horn Gf-Gc model of intelligence, or Guilford's Structure of Intellect model may shed some important light on the child's unique abilities. Using other models to explain scores should follow the same general steps outlined above. That is, the examiner might describe and define the model most suited to the test data, being careful to characterize how the pattern of scores supports the model; this step should be followed by a discussion of any subtest scores that may be incompatible with the model. Then, extra-test data

Rapid Reference 5.31

Cumulative Percentages of the AM Standardization Sample Showing Score Differences

Composite Score Difference	Recog vs. Mscr	Assoc vs. Mspn	Assoc vs. Mpro	Assoc vs. Atten	Assoc vs. Mscr	Mspn vs. Mpro	Mspn vs. Atten	Mspn vs. Mscr	Mpro vs. Atten	Mpro vs. Mscr	Atten vs. Mscr
25	10.4	15.5	14.4	18.0	3.4	0.2	16.2	3.0	14.2	3.4	14.7
24	11.2	17.8	16.2	18.3	3.6	0.2	18.0	4.1	16.2	3.6	18.0
23	12.3	20.5	17.3	20.1	4.8	0.7	19.3	4.8	17.3	4.6	18.8
22	13.3	21.6	19.1	23.4	5.0	1.1	21.9	5.5	19.3	5.0	20.1
21	14.9	23.7	21.4	24.7	6.2	1.4	23.7	6.2	21.9	5.7	23.7
20	17.9	25.5	24.1	28.0	8.0	1.8	25.0	8.4	24.2	7.3	25.8
19	19.2	28.5	27.1	32.6	8.9	2.7	26.0	10.0	26.0	9.1	27.6
18	21.3	32.1	29.2	33.9	10.7	3.9	28.1	11.6	28.6	11.8	31.2
17	25.6	34.9	33.9	36.8	13.2	5.2	31.4	14.8	32.0	14.1	32.2
16	26.9	37.6	35.8	40.9	16.9	6.4	34.8	16.4	37.1	17.8	34.5
15	30.1	39.9	38.5	42.9	20.3	8.7	38.1	19.1	40.2	20.5	39.4

Composite Score Difference	Recog vs. Mscr	Assoc vs. Mspn	Assoc vs. Mpro	Assoc vs. Atten	Assoc vs. Mscr	Mspn vs. Mpro	Mspn vs. Atten	Mspn vs. Mscr	Mpro vs. Atten	Mpro vs. Mscr	Atten vs. Mscr
14	34.1	43.1	41.2	46.3	24.1	10.9	41.2	22.3	42.5	23.7	41.8
13	35.7	46.9	44.6	53.0	28.5	14.4	45.1	26.2	45.6	27.8	45.9
12	41.1	50.1	48.5	53.2	31.0	16.4	48.5	31.2	47.4	30.8	50.5
11	44.5	54.0	51.5	59.4	35.3	20.7	51.8	35.1	50.5	37.1	52.1
10	50.7	57.9	55.6	63.5	40.8	23.2	54.6	41.9	55.2	39.9	55.2
9	54.7	60.6	61.0	65.6	45.8	26.9	58.0	44.9	59.0	46.0	59.5
8	59.5	64.2	65.1	70.4	50.1	31.7	62.1	54.2	63.7	52.4	64.2
7	65.1	67.7	71.1	74.0	58.1	36.9	67.5	61.0	68.8	56.3	69.6
6	68.3	72.0	74.3	76.6	62.2	43.5	70.1	66.3	73.5	63.6	75.8
5	73.3	74.9	79.3	83.5	68.6	52.2	74.7	72.4	77.8	69.0	78.4

Note. The AM Composite Scale full names are Recognition Memory, Memory Screener, Associative Memory, Memory Span, Memory Process, and Attention. From Roid and Miller, 1997.

Cumulative Percentages of the VR Standardization Sample Showing Score Differences

Composite Score Difference	Brief IQ vs. Spatial	Brief IQ vs. Fluid	Brief IQ vs. FundVis	FSIQ vs. Spatial	FSIQ vs. Fluid	FSIQ vs. FundVis	Spatial vs. Fluid	Fluid vs. FundVis
25	6.8	1.5	8.7	0.6	3.2	3.0	8.5	17.0
24	6.8	1.5	10.2	1.4	3.7	3.8	8.9	18.1
23	7.5	2.6	11.5	1.7	4.7	4.4	11.0	19.5
22	8.5	3.0	12.1	2.7	5.2	5.0	12.6	20.7
21	10.8	3.7	13.4	3.3	6.5	6.3	14.9	22.6
20	11.8	4.1	16.1	3.7	7.9	7.0	17.2	25.0
19	13.5	5.3	18.3	5.0	8.5	9.0	19.3	26.9
18	15.7	6.0	20.2	6.4	10.8	11.1	21.1	29.3
17	17.8	8.2	23.1	7.0	13.0	12.7	23.6	31.6
16	21.5	9.4	25.2	9.3	15.4	15.8	27.5	34.6
15	24.4	12.0	29.1	11.6	17.1	19.6	31.1	38.4
14	26.7	13.7	33.2	13.7	20.7	21.8	34.0	42.0

Composite Score Difference	Brief IQ vs. Spatial	Brief IQ vs. Fluid	Brief IQ vs. FundVis	FSIQ vs. Spatial	FSIQ vs. Fluid	FSIQ vs. FundVis	Spatial vs. Fluid	Fluid vs. FundVis
13	29.4	18.1	36.7	15.5	23.1	24.8	36.4	44.9
12	32.7	20.0	41.2	17.8	27.1	28.4	40.4	48.8
11	37.5	25.1	46.1	21.7	30.7	32.1	43.3	52.1
10	41.8	28.2	49.5	25.9	35.4	37.1	46.8	56.1
9	46.4	36.6	54.3	30.4	40.3	41.7	53.6	61.8
8	53.0	40.1	58.3	37.7	46.9	47.1	59.4	66.3
7	60.0	47.7	64.0	44.1	51.6	53.6	64.8	70.6
6	65.8	52.0	70.0	51.1	60.3	61.3	68.3	74.8
5	71.2	63.1	74.2	58.4	66.9	67.5	73.9	79.5

Note. The VR Composite Scale full names are Brief IQ Screener, Full Scale IQ (FSIQ), Fluid Reasoning Composite, Fundamental Visualization, and Spatial Visualization. From Roid and Miller, 1997.

Data and Table Copyright © 1997 by Stoelting Co. All rights reserved. Used with permission.

should be considered to either support or refute the logic of using this particular model. Finally, the examiner is obligated to discuss how this model might be applied to explain strengths and weaknesses and the relationship between those and real-world applications (e.g., educational strategies).

Step 5: Subtest Interpretation   In this stage of interpretation the focus is on individual subtests. Although significant composite or scale deviation is considered an important index of functioning, examiners should be aware that nonsignificant variability among scales does not necessarily mean that a test profile contains no significant variability. Subtest scores may yield statistically significant but offsetting differences that result in similar composite scores across scales. That is, the Fluid Reasoning and Spatial Visualization Composites may be similar, but subtests may vary significantly within and/or across the two. Therefore, the determination of whether the FSIQ is a reasonable estimate of overall cognitive functioning is not only based on composite score differences, but must also be considered at the subtest level. Of course, in situations where composites are considered useful independent of the need to obtain an FSIQ, as within the AM Battery, the same logic applies.

To evaluate subtest variability within scales the examiner may refer to Appendixes F1.3 and F2.3 in the *Leiter-R Manual*. Differences required for significance between each subtest and the mean subtest scores are provided by age level for the Brief IQ, FSIQ, and other comparisons. That is, using these data, it is possible to compare a particular subtest mean to all the subtests comprising the Brief IQ, all the subtests comprising the FSIQ, and the mean of various other sets of subtests. Those appendixes have been excerpted and are included in Rapid References 5.33 and 5.34. Also, data show difference values earned by extreme percentages of the standardization sample, notably the extreme 1%, 2%, 5%, 10%, and 25%. Examiners may use the data to make comparisons between subtests and any particular set of other subtests (e.g., seven subtests for the VR Battery, ages 11 to 20). However, it should be noted that subtests are not compared to the means of particular *composite* area subtests (e.g., Spatial Visualization, Memory Span). In some cases, such a comparison would not be possible. That is, some of the composite areas contain only two subtests (Fundamental Visualization, Memory Recognition). In those cases, it is possible to make a pairwise comparison only.

The *Leiter-R Manual* does not provide a comprehensive appendix showing differences required at various levels of significance for comparing subtest means to the means of various composites (with the exception of the com-

⟪Rapid Reference 5.33

Differences between Profile Averages and Individual VR Subtest Scaled Scores at Each Age Level—Significant Difference Values and Difference Values at Various Percentiles of the VR Standardization Sample

Cluster vs. Subtest	Sig. Diff. (.05)	Difference Values at				
		1%	2%	5%	10%	25%
All Ages: Average of Four Subtests (Brief IQ) vs.						
Figure Ground	4.36	5.3	5.0	4.0	3.5	2.5
Form Completion	3.96	6.0	5.3	4.3	3.5	2.5
Repeated Patterns	4.33	6.0	5.5	4.5	3.8	2.5
Sequential Order	4.36	5.5	5.0	4.0	3.3	2.3
Ages 2 to 5: Average of Six Subtests (Full IQ) vs.						
Figure Ground	4.76	5.5	5.0	4.3	3.5	2.5
Form Completion	4.20	6.0	5.3	4.3	3.5	2.5
Repeated Patterns	4.72	6.5	5.8	4.7	3.8	2.6
Sequential Order	4.76	5.7	5.0	4.2	3.6	2.4
Matching	4.35	5.8	5.3	4.5	3.7	2.5
Classification	4.35	5.5	4.8	4.2	3.7	2.5
Ages 6 to 20: Average of Six Subtests (Full IQ) vs.						
Figure Ground	4.85	5.5	5.0	4.3	3.5	2.5
Form Completion	4.30	6.0	5.3	4.5	3.7	2.5
Repeated Patterns	4.81	6.3	5.5	4.5	3.8	2.7
Sequential Order	4.85	5.3	5.0	4.2	3.5	2.3
Design Analogies	4.54	5.5	5.2	4.0	3.3	2.5
Paper Folding	4.72	6.3	5.5	4.7	3.8	2.5

(continued)

Cluster vs. Subtest	Sig. Diff. (.05)	Difference Values at				
		1%	2%	5%	10%	25%
Ages 2 to 5: Average of Seven Subtests vs.						
Figure Ground	4.83	5.6	5.1	4.3	3.5	2.5
Form Completion	4.21	5.9	5.3	4.4	3.5	2.5
Repeated Patterns	4.78	6.5	5.9	4.7	3.9	2.6
Sequential Order	4.83	5.8	5.1	4.3	3.6	2.4
Matching	4.38	5.7	5.3	4.4	3.6	2.4
Classification	4.38	5.6	5.0	4.1	3.7	2.6
Picture Context	4.04	5.1	4.9	4.1	3.6	2.6
Ages 11 to 20: Average of Seven Subtests vs.						
Figure Ground	4.99	5.6	5.0	4.3	3.5	2.5
Form Completion	4.39	6.0	5.5	4.5	3.7	2.5
Repeated Patterns	4.94	6.3	5.6	4.6	3.8	2.6
Sequential Order	4.99	5.5	5.0	4.1	3.5	2.4
Design Analogies	4.65	5.6	5.2	4.1	3.5	2.4
Paper Folding	4.85	6.3	5.6	4.5	3.8	2.5
Figure Rotation	4.60	6.0	5.9	4.4	3.7	2.6

Note. From Roid and Miller, 1997.

parisons shown in Rapid References 5.33 and 5.34). Consequently, we suggest that examiners use as a general rule the value of five as a criterion for making comparisons. That is, if one subtest differs from the mean of three or more subtests within a given composite area by five or more points, that particular subtest is not measuring the (composite) construct very well. Similarly, if two subtests within a composite differ by five or more points, those subtests are not measuring the same construct. In both cases, the overall composite score is not very meaningful. Based on our inspection of the Leiter-R data reported in Appendixes F1.3, F1.4, F2.3, and F2.4, we believe five points is of sufficient magnitude to meet the criteria of "statistical significance" and is rare enough

≋Rapid Reference 5.34

Differences between Profile Averages and Individual AM Subtest Scaled Scores at Each Age Level—Significant Difference Values and Difference Values at Various Percentiles of the AM Standardization Sample

Profile vs. Subtest	Sig. Diff. (.05)	Difference Values at				
		1%	2%	5%	10%	25%
Ages 2 to 3: Average of Three AM Subtests vs.						
Associated Pairs	3.98	5.3	5.0	4.0	3.5	2.3
Forward Memory	3.71	5.3	5.0	4.0	3.3	2.3
Attention Sustained	3.57	6.0	5.7	4.3	3.7	2.3
Ages 4 to 5: Average of Five AM Subtests vs.						
Associated Pairs	4.79	5.8	5.2	4.2	3.7	2.4
Immediate Recognition	4.19	5.0	4.6	4.0	3.2	2.2
Forward Memory	4.31	5.8	5.3	4.4	3.6	2.4
Attention Sustained	4.06	7.0	6.0	4.7	3.8	2.7
Delayed Recognition	4.44	5.4	4.6	4.0	3.0	2.0
Ages 6 to 10: Average of 10 AM Subtests vs.						
Associated Pairs	5.58	5.7	4.9	4.2	3.5	2.4
Immediate Recognition	4.75	6.2	5.5	4.4	3.5	2.2
Forward Memory	4.93	6.0	5.7	4.7	3.7	2.5
Attention Sustained	4.57	7.0	6.3	4.8	4.0	2.8
Reverse Memory	4.75	6.5	5.6	5.0	4.1	2.9
Visual Coding	4.69	6.1	5.7	4.9	4.0	2.9
Spatial Memory	4.75	6.9	5.6	4.7	4.0	2.9
Delayed Pairs	5.63	7.1	6.1	4.9	3.9	2.6
Delayed Recognition	5.10	6.3	4.8	4.1	3.4	2.6
Attention Divided	4.69	7.1	6.8	5.4	4.8	3.1

(continued)

Profile vs. Subtest	Sig. Diff. (.05)	Difference Values at				
		1%	2%	5%	10%	25%
Ages 11 to 20: Average of Eight AM Subtests vs.						
Associated Pairs	5.34	5.6	5.1	4.1	3.4	2.3
Forward Memory	4.74	6.1	5.6	4.5	3.7	2.5
Attention Sustained	4.40	6.9	6.0	4.8	3.9	2.7
Reverse Memory	4.57	6.6	5.9	4.8	4.0	2.8
Visual Coding	4.52	6.3	5.6	5.0	3.9	2.8
Spatial Memory	4.57	6.6	5.6	4.6	4.0	2.9
Delayed Pairs	5.38	6.6	6.1	4.8	4.0	2.6
Attention Divided	4.52	7.0	6.3	5.6	4.6	3.0

Note. From Roid and Miller, 1997.

to warrant interpretation. The rationale to accept five as general criterion is based on two considerations. First, the majority of comparisons reported in Leiter-R Appendixes F1.3 and F2.3 round to 5 (35 of 56 comparisons). Second, adopting a slightly conservative criterion helps guard against making familywise errors when making multiple comparisons.

The process of comparing individual subtest scores with the average subtest score should be completed for each composite or scale as necessary (i.e., FSIQ, Memory Span). For example, if scores between the composites are not significantly or abnormally large within the FSIQ Battery, subtests should be compared to the overall mean in a "pooled" procedure. The pooled procedure examines the extent to which individual subtests deviate from the *overall* average subtest score. The process requires that the mean of six Leiter-R subtests be computed and each subtest score be individually compared to the mean of the six to identify outliers (i.e., scores that differ by five points or more from the overall subtest mean). Importantly, outliers may not be interpreted as measures of a unique ability unless they have adequate subtest specificity, that is, at least 25% of the subtest variance is unique (as opposed to "common") and the unique variance is greater than error. To determine whether individual subtests

Common, Specific, and Error Variance for Leiter-R Subtests for Three Ages

Subtest	Ages 2 to 5			Ages 6 to 10			Ages 11 to 20		
	C	S	E	C	S	E	C	S	E
FG	42	33	25	59	18	23	30	44	26
DA	—	—	—	40	44	16	46	35	19
FC	54	36	10	52	36	12	39	45	16
M	43	50	07	42	31	27	—	—	—
SO	30	42	28	46	34	20	62	08	30
RP	40	40	20	40	34	16	45	30	25
PC	33	47	20	—	—	—	—	—	—
C	46	38	16	—	—	—	—	—	—
PF	—	—	—	13	58	28	68	13	19
FR	—	—	—	—	—	—	40	42	18
AP	40	35	25	72	0	28	94	0	06
IR	—	—	—	62	20	18	—	—	—
FM	45	42	13	51	28	21	44	32	24
AS	59	24	17	23	60	17	25	67	08
RM	—	—	—	49	36	15	34	49	17
VC	—	—	—	46	43	11	37	42	21
SM	—	—	—	36	46	18	42	44	14
DP	—	—	—	62	08	30	50	16	34
DR	—	—	—	89	0	11	—	—	—
AD	—	—	—	23	45	32	11	55	34

Note. FG = Figure Ground; DA = Design Analogies; FC = Form Completion; M = Matching; SO = Sequential Order; RP = Repeated Patterns; PC = Picture Context; C = Classification; PF = Paper Folding; FR = Figure Rotation; AP = Associated Pairs; IR = Immediate Recognition; FM = Forward Memory; AS = Attention Sustained; RM = Reverse Memory; VC = Visual Coding; SM = Spatial Memory; DP = Delayed Pairs; DR = Delayed Recognition; AD = Attention Divided. Decimals omitted. C = Common Variance; S = Specific Variance; E = Error Variance. From Roid and Miller, 1997.

Rapid Reference 5.36

Cognitive Processes Underlying Performance on the Leiter-R Subtests

Abilities	Visualization and Reasoning Battery Subtests									
	FG	DA	FC	M	SO	RP	PC	C	PF	FR
Reasoning										
Deductive Reasoning	X		X	X			X		X	X
Abstraction/Inductive Reasoning		X			X	X		X		
Categories/Sorting		X					X	X		
Analogies/Relationships		X								
Generating Rules and Understanding Relationships		X			X	X	X	X		
Part to Whole Relationships	X		X	X			X	X	X	
Perceptual Organization			X					X		X
Sequential Information					X	X				
Pattern Recognition		X				X		X		
Contextual Knowledge	X						X	X		
Visualization										
Scanning Search	X		X	X			X			
Visual-Spatial		X							X	
Discrimination/Recognition	X		X	X						X

Visualization and Reasoning Battery Subtests

Abilities	FG	DA	FC	M	SO	RP	PC	C	PF	FR
Visual Neglect		X								
Closure	X						X			
Memory										
Immediate										
Delayed-Long Term										
Retention Span-Short Term Memory										
Working			X			X	X			
Attention										
To Detail	X									
To Simultaneous Stimuli				X			X		X	X
Sustained/Span	X									
Distractibility	X									
Processing Style										
Flexibility/Shifting	X							X	X	
Interference Task	X									
Impulsivity/Inhibition	X	X		X	X	X			X	X
Organization	X	X					X			
Fine Motor-Pencil Grasp										

Note. FG = Figure Ground; DA = Design Analogies; FC = Form Completion; M = Matching; SO = Sequential Order; RP = Repeated Patterns; PC = Picture Context; C = Classification; PF = Paper Folding; FR = Figure Rotation. From Roid and Miller, 1997.

Rapid Reference 5.37

Cognitive Processes Underlying Performance on the Leiter-R Subtests

Abilities	AP	IR	FM	AS	RM	VC	SM	DP	DR	AD
Reasoning										
Deductive Reasoning										
Abstraction/Inductive Reasoning						X				
Categories/Sorting										
Analogies/Relationships						X				
Generating Rules and Understanding Relationships						X				
Part to Whole Relationships										
Perceptual Organization			X							
Sequential Information					X					
Pattern Recognition										
Contextual Knowledge										X
Visualization										
Scanning/Search				X						
Visual-Spatial										
Discrimination/Recognition		X					X			
Visual Neglect				X			X			
Closure										

Attention and Memory Battery

Abilities	AP	IR	FM	AS	RM	VC	SM	DP	DR	AD
Memory										
Immediate	×	×								
Delayed-Long Term						×	×	×	×	
Retention Span–Short Term Memory			×		×		×			
Working					×	×	×			×
Attention										
To Detail	×	×		×						
To Simultaneous Stimuli				×	×	×	×	×		×
Sustained/Span			×	×	×	×	×			
Distractibility				×	×					×
Processing Style										
Flexibility/Shifting				×		×				×
Interference Task			×	×	×		×			×
Impulsivity/Inhibition			×	×	×	×				×
Organization				×		×				×
Fine Motor–Pencil Grasp				×						

Note. AP = Associated Pairs; IR = Immediate Recognition; FM = Forward Memory; AS = Attention Sustained; RM = Reverse Memory; VC = Visual Coding; SM = Spatial Memory; DP = Delayed Pairs; DR = Delayed Recognition; AD = Attention Divided. From Roid and Miller, 1997.

possess sufficient specificity to be interpreted as measuring some unique cognitive ability, refer to Rapid Reference 5.35. If subtests have sufficient variance for interpretation, consider the abilities that underpin individual subtests in Rapid Reference 5.36 and 5.37.

This information will help the examiner begin to generate hypotheses or potential explanations for individual subtest strengths and weaknesses (e.g., conflicting subtest scores, inconsistent subtest patterns). Importantly, it is necessary to reconcile strong and weak abilities by examining comparable abilities assessed by other subtests administered in the battery. Finally, examiners should consider additional extra-test variables, such as the referral problem, teacher/parent reports, class and assessment behavioral observations, and students' work samples to support or refute hypotheses that are generated during the interpretation process.

These same guidelines can be followed for determining strengths and weaknesses for any composite. For example, any subtest can be compared to its scale mean (i.e., Visual Coding to the three Memory Process subtests). The strategy is the same.

Step 6: Generate Hypotheses about Fluctuation in the Leiter-R Profile If scores are consistent with the test model (i.e., they show little variability, or they show clear, significant, and rare Fluid Reasoning versus Spatial Visualization or Memory Process versus Associative Memory differences), interpretation is straightforward and simple. However, such patterns are not particularly common and other models may be investigated (e.g., simultaneous versus successive, Gf-Gc). Moreover, in some cases no model-based approach will explain functioning, and individual subtest scores must be examined. In order to facilitate generation of hypotheses about strengths and weaknesses it will be helpful to refer again to Rapid References 5.36 and 5.37. In addition, refer to the general descriptions of the abilities assessed by the composites in the early portion of this chapter. Obviously, reading the background in the *Leiter-R Manual* will be useful.

In some instances, hypotheses may be generated because of unique features of the test. Certain features of the Leiter-R are particularly important to consider because of the relevance of these features to interpretation. *First,* the Leiter-R is administered primarily through the use of gestures and demonstration; consequently, only indirect hypotheses can be generated from test performance about the examinee's verbal skills. The examiner will have some knowledge of the student's verbal abilities from extra-test sources and these skills should be described in the background section of the report. *Second,* the test allows the opportunity for both motoric (e.g., card movement) and non-motoric-reduced (e.g., pointing) responses. Administration of the subtests can be modified so that only a pointing response will be required on many of the subtests. The use of motoric and motor-reduced subtests facilitates administration by optimizing motivation and rapport. For example, a very shy child may be encouraged initially to point in response to items, and later, as better rapport is gained, other, more motorically involved responses may be possible. *Third,* because the Leiter-R offers two versions in order to obtain an IQ, administration time can be controlled by the examiner, depending on the number of subtests administered. Also, additional subtests from either the VR or the AM battery may be administered at the examiner's discretion. The examiner should describe in the psychological report the rationale for choosing a particular version of the test.

Importantly, there are a few suggested pairwise comparisons possible from the so-called Special Diagnostic Subtests (Roid & Miller, 1997), as described in the *Leiter-R Manual.* These comparisons are taken from the AM Battery only and include: Associated Pairs: Familiar versus Random; Delayed Pairs: Familiar versus Random; Visual Coding: Standard Profile Score versus Upper Range; and Attention Divided: Pictures Correctly Identified versus Cards Sorted. The strategies for making these clinical comparisons are described in the *Leiter-R Manual.*

Finally, data from the four rating scales (Self, Parent, Teacher, Examiner) may be helpful in some cases. In particular, these data can help test hypotheses developed from use of the standard scores, build context, identify problems and/or resources, and so forth.

Summary of Interpretive Steps

The Test Model interpretive process relies on interpreting a multidimensional test according to the theoretical model that underpins the development of the test. For example, based on his clinical experience, Wechsler believed that human cognitive performance could be categorized parsimoniously into a dichotomous verbal/nonverbal fashion (Wechsler, 1939). For some children such a dichotomy works well, and the rational-intuitive model explains their cognitive functioning accurately. Similarly, the Leiter-R Fluid Reasoning versus Spatial Visualization dichotomy may provide a parsimonious explanation for some examinees' intellectual abilities; other examinees' scores may conform nicely to an IQ versus Memory Process split. In other cases, none of the Leiter-R composite scores or patterns explain the examinees' abilities. In such cases, the application of other theoretical orientations may be helpful for understanding the student's abilities.

The primary Leiter-R scale, the VR Battery, is the one designed to provide an IQ score. Other composites are available from both the VR and AM Batteries. For most purposes examiners will compute the FSIQ and use that scale to make comparisons (FSIQ versus Memory Process; FSIQ versus Fluid Reasoning). Other composite scores can be obtained and comparisons generated (Fluid Reasoning versus Spatial Visualization; Associative Memory versus Attention). Remember that differences must be statistically significant and rare, and scatter should be appropriately low to interpret composite differences cleanly.

Next, it may be necessary to examine subtest strengths and weaknesses. Subtest scores can be compared to their scale mean (e.g., memory) or the mean of several other subtests as needed. Also, pairwise comparisons may be made. If there are statistically significant and abnormally large difference between composites, and the scatter within scales is not abnormally large, scale means should be used. If not, the overall or "pooled" mean should be used.

Finally, use task analyses to determine subtest abilities, to consider the unique skills that underlie each subtest, and to reconcile any apparent inconsistencies that might exist. Obviously, abilities measured by subtests that are designated as strengths should be eliminated as strengths if they are also abilities that are assessed by other subtests as weak. Determine the relevance of intrasubtest scatter characteristics. For example, some examinees fail easy items but pass more difficult ones, which may be indicative of educational problems such as attentional deficits or learning disabilities. Consider educational and psychological ramifications of identified strengths and weaknesses (e.g., high memory/low reasoning).

Consider intervention strategies that might remediate or accommodate identified weaknesses. When possible, the examiner should link the test results to specific to-be-learned classroom skills (e.g., calculation of addition problems) rather than attempt to remediate hypothetical constructs such as "reasoning" or "memory." It may be helpful to use the abilities assessed by the subtests as presented in the Growth Curve Record Forms. Abilities may be identified by using the Growth Curve metric or by using the rough but more easily understood age equivalents scores.

Current practice and state regulations dictate that intelligence tests scores not be used in isolation. Critics such as McDermott et al. (1990) have failed to examine the clinical value of subtest analysis when it is employed as only one bit of data that is confirmed or refuted through other data sources. Thus, we recommend that Leiter-R subtest analysis be conducted to generate hypotheses about children's unique intellectual strengths and weaknesses, but *never* without additional extra-test information that will allow the examiner to further evaluate the hypotheses that are generated. Our Appendix B provides a worksheet for quick interpretation.

SUMMARY

The Leiter-R is a colorful, multitask instrument for ages 2 through 20 years. In general, the reliabilities are adequate at the composite level, but are occasionally problematic at the subtest level, according to criteria established by Bracken (1987) and reported in Bracken and McCallum (1998). Although the test is largely nonverbal in its administration, the Leiter-R requires some verbalization and includes an array of gestures and pantomimed instructions that are vast in number and seem vague or confusing at times. The Leiter-R appears to have adequate reliability at the scale level for an instrument intended for important decision-making (Bracken, 1987, 1988; Nunnally & Bernstein, 1994). The test is composed of subtests that predominately are rated as fair or poor measures of *g*. The instrument matches proposed four- or five-factor theoretical underpinnings fairly well, with some minor model variation across the age levels. When used with individuals who have recently immigrated to the United States, practitioners should be aware that some Leiter-R subtests contain stimulus materials that are influenced considerably by Western culture. Administration is accomplished in a nearly completely nonverbal fashion. However, the directions sometimes seem vague and they permit examiners to interact verbally to provide clarification and elaboration during test administration in some cases. Interpretation may be facilitated by following guidelines used by experts in the field and adapted and reported in this chapter, as a means of examining performance from the molar to molecular level.

🔖 TEST YOURSELF 🔖

1. **Which one of the following subtests is included on the Fluid Reasoning Scale?**
   - (a) Matching
   - (b) Paper Folding
   - (c) Classification
   - (d) Repeated Patterns

2. **The Leiter-R is based on what theory?**
   - (a) Jensen's Level I (memory) and II (reasoning), with g at the apex
   - (b) Gardner's Multiple Intelligences
   - (c) Thurstone's Primary Abilities
   - (d) Hierarchical g, with Gc, Gf, Gv

3. **Which nonverbal test was standardized using NO language?**
   - (a) Leiter-R
   - (b) Columbia
   - (c) WISC-III Performance Scale
   - (d) UNIT

4. **The Leiter-R is designed for examinees ages**
   - (a) 2 years to 20 years, 11 months
   - (b) 5 years to 21 years, 11 months
   - (c) 5 years to 19 years, 11 months
   - (d) 5 years to 17 years, 11 months

5. **An abnormally large and rare discrepancy between FR and SV means the discrepancy**
   - (a) Occurs in the extreme 5% of the population
   - (b) Occurs in the extreme 10% of the population
   - (c) Occurs in the extreme 15% of the population
   - (d) Is equivalent to a statistically significant discrepancy

6. **The Leiter-R yields which of the following Global Scores?**
   - (a) Auditory processing
   - (b) Visual processing
   - (c) Brief IQ
   - (d) Long-term Memory Quotient

7. Which of the Leiter-R subtests taps the ability to sequence information?

(a) Repeated Patterns

(b) Cube Design

(c) Matching

(d) Figure Ground

8. Which of the Leiter-R subtests taps the ability to assess working memory?

(a) Figure Ground

(b) Cube Design

(c) Associated Pairs

(d) Reverse Memory

9. Which one of the Leiter-R subtests produces the poorest estimate of internal consistency reliability (averaged across ages)?

(a) Attention Divided

(b) Forward Memory

(c) Spatial Memory

(d) Immediate Recognition

10. The *Leiter-R Manual* recommends (and reports) using the _____ level of statistical significance to determine composite differences.

(a) .01

(b) .05

(c) .10

(d) .15

Answers: 1. d; 2. d; 3. d; 4. a; 5. c; 6. c; 7. a; 8. d; 9. a; 10. b

Six

MULTIDIMENSIONAL NONVERBAL INTELLIGENCE TESTS: STRENGTHS, WEAKNESSES, AND CLINICAL APPLICATIONS OF THE LEITER-R

The Leiter-R offers a number of strengths; in addition, it has some salient weakness. Based on our use of the test, examination of the *Leiter-R Manual* and the test materials, and feedback from users around the country, we have obtained considerable information regarding the test's strengths and weaknesses. For example, we know that the test, with two batteries and four rating scales, offers assessment of many constructs and is useful for children as young as 2 years of age and as old as 20 years, 11 months. The test offers several administration options, ranging from a relatively short four-subtest version to a much longer version which can be "tailor-made" by the examiner. The Leiter-R has 20 subtests in all, ten in each of two batteries, although not all are appropriate for all ages. In addition, there are four rating scales available; these rating scales may be completed by the examinee, the examiner, the examinee's parent, and the examinee's teacher. The scales provide information about the examinee's attention, impulse control and organization, social skills, mood, energy level, self-esteem, and ability to adapt. Also, we are aware of some weaknesses, including problems with the standardization sample (e.g., underrepresentation at certain ages for some subtests), cumbersome administration directions, floor and ceiling limitations, and poor representation for some populations in some of the validity studies.

In this chapter we present specific strengths and weaknesses, grouped into the following categories: test development, administration and scoring, standardization, reliability and validity, and interpretation. We follow our discussion of strengths and weaknesses by mentioning several test development characteristics designed to ensure fairness.

TEST DEVELOPMENT/STANDARDIZATION
STRENGTHS AND WEAKNESSES

The Leiter-R adopts as its theoretical base a rather complex model, consistent with the research of Gustafsson (1984) and Carroll (1993), both of whom consider intelligence to be hierarchically structured and multifaceted. The Leiter-R model presumes a multifaceted arrangement with general intelligence at the apex and several broad but subordinate factors at a second level, including visualization, attention, reasoning, memory, and so forth. Subordinate to these general factors are the specific abilities operationalized by the subtests, such as sustained attention, forward memory, and figure-ground relationships.

The model represents a strength because of its reliance on empirical literature. In fact, Roid and Miller (1997) define intelligence as measured by the Leiter-R as "operational and empirical rather than theoretical," and as characterized by "the general ability to perform complex nonverbal mental manipulations, related to conceptualization, inductive reasoning, and visualization" (p. 103). It should be noted that the empirical fit, as defined by factor analytic data, is not exact. That is, the factorial structure varies slightly as a function of age and is not entirely consistent with the global-score arrangement. In addition, the standardization data are somewhat problematic. For example, only about one-third of the examinees were administered both Visualization and Reasoning (VR) *and* Attention and Memory (AM) Batteries. Also, the sample size is somewhat small in general and, for some ages, much too small. The VR Battery was standardized on 1,719 children and the AM Battery on 763 children. Overall, the VR Battery is based on a sample size of slightly fewer than 100 individuals per age level. In addition, for the seven-year age span from 14 through 20, there is an average of only 41 examinees per age. The AM Battery includes fewer than 100 examinees at every age across the entire age range, with samples ranging from a low of 42 examinees at some age levels (i.e., 7, 8, 11, and 18 to 29) to a high of 86 children at the 2-year level. These samples may produce unstable normative data.

In general, the VR Battery normative sample matches the U.S. population fairly well on most strata (e.g., gender, race, socioeconomic status, community size, and geographic region), though the number and location of specific sites are not reported. Although the overall match to the U.S. population is within about 2% on relevant variables, there is over- and underrepresentation for specific variables from as much as 6 to 8 percent. For example, only 60.2% of the 10-year-old children in the sample are Caucasian, compared with 68.4% in the population. Gender representation is similarly problematic, showing VR norms for males ranging from 46.7% to 54.8%, depending on age. The AM sample shows even larger discrepancies in relation to the population. For example, only 39.6% of the sample is male for ages 14 to 15, while 64.6% is male for age 3. Similar discrepancies exist for the parent education level variable. The percentage in the "Less than High School" category ranges from 2.3% at age 6 to 26.7% at age 2, compared with the national average of 19.8%.

Development of the Leiter-R was guided by four primary rationales (Roid & Miller, 1997). These rationales are described in detail in the *Leiter-R Manual* and are mentioned briefly here. The rationales include: (a) the need to develop a test to identify early cognitive delays; (b) the need to assess small increments of ability; (c) the need to build a reliable and valid scale regardless of language or motor ability; and (d) the need to assess individual's ability to transition into the work world. See Rapid Reference 6.1 for specific strengths and weaknesses.

STRENGTHS AND WEAKNESSES OF ADMINISTRATION AND SCORING

The *Leiter-R Manual* contains details of administration and scoring and the examiner must read those directions carefully. Details of administration vary considerably by subtest, even though there is an effort to ensure some consistency in the format. That is, for many of the subtests examinees are expected to indicate the correct answer by selecting or pointing to cards placed before them. The card may be placed into correct "slots" on an easel tray. The examiner is allowed to use a variety of nonverbal directions, including gestures, pointing, pantomime, and modeling. On a few subtests the examiner may use words or very short phrases to communicate time requirements and/or task demands. The nonverbal gestures and pantomime directions are provided for each subtest, and in some cases are unique to particular subtests. Thus, there is no standard set of gestures used throughout, which may limit the ease of administration across subtests. In addition, some directions require that the examiner improvise. For example, there are a number of directions such as "encourage the child to imitate you; indicate nonverbally that each pair goes

≡ Rapid Reference 6.1

Strengths and Weaknesses of Leiter-R Development/Standardization

Strengths

- The Leiter-R retained the administration format of the original Leiter in general, allowing some positive transfer of administration skills.
- Subtest selection was guided by theoretical considerations and by the need to assess young children as well as those preparing to enter the work force, the need to assess small increments of progress, and the need to provide a reliable and valid measure of abilities regardless of language.
- Because the Rasch Model was used to select items within subtests it was possible to develop "Growth Scale scores"; these scores allow direct comparison of mastery across all ages using a common metric, ranging from 380 to 560, with scores centered on beginning 5th grade (10 years, 4 months) performance.
- The Leiter-R produces a standard score psychometric scale such that the mean is set to 100 and the standard deviation to 15 for global scores and to 10 and 3 for subtests, to ease cross-battery comparisons.
- The stimulus materials are colorful and attractive for children.

Weaknesses

- Not all subtests extend across the entire age range; in fact, only 7 of 20 extend across the entire range.
- The factor analytic data fail to fit exactly the theoretical structure as depicted by the global scores; that is, the factor structure varies slightly as a function of age although the overall global score arrangement does not vary.
- The standardization sample is problematic in that only about one-third of the examinees were administered both Visualization and Reasoning *and* Attention and Memory batteries, limiting direct comparisons somewhat.
- The standardization was somewhat small compared to other major, individually-administered intelligence tests, and was under- or overrepresented on various stratification variables, depending on age and battery.

together; indicate that the child should point to the red apple only." The authors note that in some cases it may be necessary for the examiner to "create unusual methods by which the child can communicate their answers" (p. 76). They suggest that the examiner should "Feel free to extrapolate and invent your own ways of communicating nonverbally what is expected of the child being tested" (p. 21). Fortunately, the Leiter-R authors appreciate the fact that test adaptation may affect scores and note that the norms may be changed by these adaptations. Unfortunately, there is no way to determine how much the norms are affected by such idiosyncratic changes and, as a result, how much error may be introduced into the scoring process.

The Leiter-R offers a variety of administration options. It is possible to obtain a Full Scale IQ by administering six subtests from the VR Battery; a Brief IQ can be obtained by administering only four subtests. Other VR global scores may be obtained (i.e., Fluid Reasoning, Fundamental Visualization, Spatial Visualization). In addition, several global scores may be obtained from the AM Battery, including Memory Screening, Associative Memory, Memory Span, Attention, Memory Process, and Recognition Memory formats; an Abbreviated Battery; a Standard Battery; and an Extended Battery. Importantly, not all global scores are available for all ages. These formats allow for considerable flexibility.

Scoring is facilitated in some cases by the test booklet and *Manual* formats; however, these materials contain some salient weaknesses as well. The record books are clear and inclusive; they offer the examiner space to plot raw-to-scale score transformations, age equivalents, Growth Scale scores, and profiles for standard scores and item-to-Growth Scale score transformations. However, the correct answers are not on the record booklets, nor do the booklets offer work space to test hypotheses (e.g., identifying subtest strengths and weaknesses or determining the statistical significance of global score differences). Moreover, the booklets do not contain start and stop rules for subtest administration. The *Manual* is arranged such that transformations from raw to standard scores are straightforward, but the process is made somewhat difficult by the need to refer to multiple tables to obtain essential score information. For example, raw score to scale score transformations for subtests are found on page A-6 for a 3 year, 10 month old child; the sum of the scaled score can be translated to a Brief IQ on page D-2, but it is necessary to turn to page K-1 to find the percentile rank. Finally, the standard error of measurement is found in another table on page 104.

Stimulus materials are provided on three easels, which contain stimulus plates, directions, and scoring information. The four Rating Scales are easily administered and scored, and the scales have many of the necessary directions printed on them. Finally, a computer scoring system is available. Specific administration and scoring strengths and weaknesses are shown in Rapid Reference 6.2.

STRENGTHS AND WEAKNESSES OF LEITER-R TECHNICAL PROPERTIES

The *Leiter-R Manual* describes data addressing the reliability and validity of the test. To determine internal consistency, coefficient alphas are reported. Average coefficient alphas for the VR subtests range from .75 to .90, depending on age. Average coefficient alphas for the AM subtests are generally lower, ranging from .67 to .87. Composite reliabilities for the VR Battery range from .88 to .93. Full Scale reliabilities range from .91 to .93. Global score reliabilities from the AM Battery range from .75 to .93.

Stability coefficients are also reported. For the VR Battery, stability coefficients range from .61 to .81 for subtests, and from .83 to .90 for global or composite scores. In general, coefficients are higher for older children than for younger children, as would be expected. For example, the range for subtest scores for ages 2 through 7 is .61 to .81; for ages 11 to 20, .65 to .90. No intertest interval was reported in the *Manual*. Importantly, these scores may be inflated due to significant expansion in variability of scores. Every subtest and global score reported in the stability study show standard score estimates of variability (i.e., standard deviations) that are much greater than their respective normative standard deviations. For example, the standard deviation for the FSIQ is reported to be 30 for ages 11 to 20, which is two times the normative standard deviation of 15. The *Leiter-R Manual* reports only corrected values; both corrected and uncorrected values should have been reported to aid the examiner in determining the significance of the expansion in variability problems.

In addition to the correlation coefficients, the *Leiter-R Manual* also reports mean score differences for subtests and global scores across the test-retest interval. Gains are variable, ranging from only .10 standard deviation to 1.4 standard deviations. Global score gains range from around .33 to .50 standard

Rapid Reference 6.2

Strengths and Weaknesses of Leiter-R Administration and Scoring

Strengths

- Administration of the Leiter-R is almost language free; that is, most subtests can be administered without language.
- The record forms are user-friendly, and include space for making relevant raw-to-standard score transformation easily.
- There are a variety of administration formats depending on available time and need. A Brief IQ, which can be obtained by administering four subtests, is useful for screening; the Full Scale IQ may be obtained by administering six subtests and is more appropriate for providing scores for routine placement decisions.
- Three VR global scores may be obtained (i.e., Fluid Reasoning, Fundamental Visualization, and Spatial Visualization).
- The AM Battery offers several global scores, including Memory Screening, Associative Memory, Memory Span, Attention, Memory Process, and Recognition Memory.
- The Manual and the easels offer administration directions; scoring criteria are provided on the easels.
- In general, items are scored dichotomously.
- A computerized scoring system is available.

Weaknesses

- The Manual does not show the gestures used in the standardization of the Leiter-R, nor does it show placement of the stimulus materials and the appropriate seating arrangement.
- On some subtests, administration and scoring is cumbersome or confusing. For example, the Sustained Attention subtest uses three booklets, a scoring template, and several steps to obtain an "adjusted correct" score; the Attention Divided subtest requires that the examinee perform two operations at once and he or she may earn two scores on each item.
- There is little standardization of discontinue criteria across subtests.
- The Manual encourages use of various strategies and techniques to communicate and urges idiosyncratic administration adaptations, which may increase scoring error.
- Information needed to obtain raw-to-scale score transformations is located in multiple tables in various sections of the Manual.

deviations. Because the interval is not reported it is difficult to make sense of the gain scores.

For the AM Battery, corrected test-retest coefficients range from .55 to .85 for a small sample of 45 examinees ranging in age from 6 to 17 years (median age, 10 years, 11 months). Corrected subtest stability coefficients range from .55 to .85; global score coefficients range from .61 to .85. Practice effects show average gains of about .50 standard deviations. Again the interval is not reported.

Reliability estimates for the subtests of the four rating scales are typically higher than for the VR and AM Batteries. Reliabilities are typically in the .80s and .90s for those subtests. (See page 158 of the *Leiter-R Manual.*)

According to the *Leiter-R Manual,* data from 11 validity studies provide evidence that the instrument can discriminate among special groups (i.e., speech/language impaired; hearing impaired; traumatic brain injured; motor delayed; cognitively delayed; Attention-Deficit/Hyperactivity Disordered; gifted; nonverbal learning disabled; verbal learning disabled; English as a second language, Spanish; English as a second language, Asian or other). The mean scores are reported in tables in the *Leiter-R Manual.* Some of the scores are consistent with expectations. For example, the cognitively delayed sample means range from 55.4 to 67.1 across age and type of score (i.e., Brief IQ or FSIQ). However, in general, the mean scores seemed lower than would be expected. With the exception of the gifted sample, all earned means below 100 on every possible IQ and composite score, and many of the composites were in the 70s, and 80s. For children ages 6 to 20, the gifted sample earned a mean FSIQ of 114.6 and all special groups earned mean FSIQs of less than 90, except the two ESL groups. Means for the AM Battery are generally higher for these special populations, typically in the 80s, 90s, and low 100s.

Concurrent validity studies also are reported in the *Leiter-R Manual,* and include comparisons of the Leiter-R with other intelligence tests, such as the original Leiter, the WISC-III, and selected subtests from the Stanford-Binet Intelligence Scale–Fourth Edition (Thorndike, Hagen, & Sattler, 1986). The correlation between the original Leiter and the Leiter-R IQ is .85. The average correlation between the Leiter-R FSIQ and WISC-III FSIQ for a sample of normative, cognitively delayed, gifted, and ESL-Spanish cases is reported in the *Examiner's Manual* as .86. It should be noted that the standard deviations on the instruments employed in these studies are higher than their corresponding normative values, ranging between 23 and 27.4 IQ points. These expanded ranges of variability can produce an inflated and misleading validity coefficient between these two instruments.

Several studies comparing the Leiter-R Brief IQ and FSIQs with various memory scales and achievement measures are reported in the *Manual;* all report small sample sizes (i.e., *n*'s of 17 to 33 subjects). These studies yield moderate to strong correlations (e.g., typically .40s to .80s) between the Leiter-R Brief IQ and FSIQ.

Construct validity was investigated by examining the factor structure of the test. The authors report support for the proposed underlying hierarchical *g* model that was used to design the instrument. However, the *g* loadings for the subtests appear to be smaller than the criterion suggested by Kaufman's (1979, 1994) for a rating of Good (> .70) for most of the subtests. In fact, all of the Leiter-R subtests are classified as either Fair (.50 to .69) or Poor (> .49) measures of *g,* except two. At ages 2 to 5 years, the Leiter-R *g* loadings range from .26 to .66, with a median of .595; *g* loadings range from .26 to .65 at ages 6 to 10 years (median = .45); and at ages 11 to 20 years, the *g* loadings range from .24 to .70, with a median of .56 (Roid & Miller, 1997, p. 192). The two subtests that qualify as Good *g*-loaders (i.e., Sequential Order and Paper Folding) meet Kaufman's criterion at only one of the three broad age levels studied (i.e., ages 11 to 20 years). As with the remaining 18 subtests, these two latter subtests were classified as Fair or Poor measures of *g* at the remaining age levels.

Additional exploratory and confirmatory factor analyses reported in the *Leiter-R Manual* provide evidence for a reasonably good fit between a proposed four- or five-factor model. However, these "fits" may or may not correspond to the global or composite score arrangement designed by the authors, depending on age. In addition, given that the Leiter-R is founded on a two battery model, one might reasonably anticipate a two-factor fit; however, such a parsimonious theoretical model and the data do not match. The model fit is fairly consistent across the age span, with support for a four-factor model at the younger age levels (i.e., ages 2 to 5 years) and a five-factor model from ages 6 through 20 years. The factors identified by the authors vary slightly in name and subtest composition across the age levels, but include such proposed abilities as Fluid Reasoning/Reasoning, Visualization/Visual Spatial, Attention, Recognition Memory, and Associative/Memory Span.

Content/construct validity was determined in part by examining growth curves. Children become more cognitively sophisticated as they age; hence, their raw scores should increase with age. In the case of the Leiter-R, Growth Scale curves should maintain the age-dependent relationship between cognitive sophistication and age, and the *Leiter-R Manual* shows consistent Growth Scale score gains as a function of age (p. 183).

In order to establish validity it is important for experts to evaluate the nature of test content. Nonverbal tests should be relatively free from cultural content. As part of a cross-battery approach to test interpretation, McGrew and Flanagan (1998) examined the prominence of cultural content embedded in various intelligence tests. McGrew and Flanagan classified nine of the 20 Leiter-R subtests as containing high levels of cultural content (i.e., Classification, Picture Context, Form Completion, Immediate Recognition, Forward Memory, Figure Ground, Delayed Recognition, Associated Pairs, and Delayed Pairs), primarily because these subtests use pictures of culture-specific objects. Three additional subtests were designated as having moderate levels of cultural content (i.e., Visual Coding, Matching, and Attention Sustained). These subtests may be of limited value when evaluating a child from another culture, depending on the particular referral problem and the background of the examinee.

Floor and ceiling data can be obtained from the tables in the *Leiter-R Manual*. Examiners should be wary that some subtests show problematic floors and ceilings at extreme ages. For example, for the VR Battery, the table in Appendix A of the *Leiter-R Manual* shows that a raw score of one point will earn scaled scores of 4 (Figure Ground), 7 (Form Completion), 5 (Matching), 8 (Sequential Order), 9 (Repeated Patterns), 6 (Picture Context), and 7 (Classification) for children ages 2 years, 0 months to 2 years, 1 month. Obviously, young cognitively limited children will not be assessed with sufficient sensitivity at this age. Only later (e.g., in the 3-year range) do scores show acceptable sensitivity. Similar scores are possible for most of the 2-year age range. A similar situation exists for the AM Battery. Of course, the problem is less severe if global scores are used.

The ceiling is somewhat problematic also. For example, maximum scores on Repeated Patterns and Form Completion for the oldest age range yield a scaled score of only 13. Similarly, the AM Battery contains a couple of problematic subtests as well. Ceilings are better when global scores are considered. For the most part, item gradients are good, particularly for global scores. See Rapid Reference 6.3 for technical strengths and weaknesses.

Rapid Reference 6.3

Strengths and Weaknesses of Leiter-R Technical Properties

Strengths

- Split-half reliability coefficients and standard errors of measurement are good for the global scores, including the Brief IQ and the Full Scale IQ (.91 to .93), and most composite scores, ranging from .75 to .93 across both batteries.

- Across all age groups, 6 of the 10 AV Battery subtests yielded average reliability coefficients above .80 (Standard Battery); four were in the .70s; six of the AM subtests also averaged .80 or better. Reliabilities for the Rating Scale subtests were higher, in general; many were in the .90s across the four rating scales (see p. 158 in the Leiter-R Manual).

- Practice effects are reported by subtest; they range from .10 to 1.40 standard deviations for subtests. Global scores gains ranged from about .33 to .50 standard deviation units.

Weaknesses

- Only corrected correlation coefficients are reported, rather than the actual coefficients, for several reliability and validity studies.

- Many subtests yielded average subtest reliabilities below .80 (see pages 156 and 157 in the Leiter-R Manual).

- Test-retest interval was not reported for the stability study in the Leiter-R Manual.

- Test-retest reliability coefficients are below the split-half values, in the main; for the composite scores coefficients ranged from .55 to .96 across both batteries.

- The specific variance for several subtest is less than 25%, making them uninterpretable as a measure of some unique ability (see Chapter 5 in this volume or p. 193 in the Leiter-R Manual).

Strengths

- Factor analytic data yield some support for the Leiter-R model. Typically four or five factors are identified that correspond roughly to the authors' suggested categories. However, there is not an exact match between factors and the theoretical arrangement of the subtests. In addition, only two of the 20 subtests (Sequential Order and Paper Folding) yield a g loading of .70 or better, a value considered good by Kaufman (1999); these values fail to support strongly the assertion that the Leiter-R provides a good measure of g.

- The *Leiter-R Manual* reports results of a number of concurrent validity studies with various measures of intelligence for different populations. Correlation coefficients showing the relationship between Leiter-R IQs and full scale scores from other major intelligence tests (e.g., Wechsler scales) are typically in the .70 to .80 range.

- The *Leiter-R Manual* reports correlations between Leiter-R scores and those from a variety of achievement tests; typically, coefficients typically range from .62 to .79. However, the sample sizes are very small, ranging from 17 to 33.

- Specific variance values are sufficient for many subtests (see Chapter 5 in this volume, or p. 193 in the *Leiter-R Manual*).

Weaknesses

- Because the floor is inadequate for cognitively limited 2-year-old examinees, cautious interpretation is advised.

CLINICAL APPLICATIONS OF THE LEITER-R

As stated in the opening remarks of Chapter 1 of the Leiter-R manual, the test was developed to provide a nonverbal measure of intellectual ability, memory, and attention that could be used to assess examinees who could not be reliably and validly assessed with traditional tests. Specific target groups identified includes those with significant communication disorders, cognitive delay, English as a second language, hearing impairments, motor impairments, traumatic brain injury, attention-deficit disorder, and certain types of learning disabilities.

In order to support the use of the Leiter-R for individuals within these groups, several studies are reported in the manual. For example, using a sample of over 724 students, 40 of whom were previously diagnosed as retarded, the authors conclude that using a cutpoint of 70 on the FSIQ yielded an overall hit rate of 96%, with correct classification of over 80% of the cognitive-delay sample, and low rates of false negative and false positive errors. For a group of previously identified gifted students, the hit rate was lower for the FSIQ (85%) using a cutpoint of *120* (compared to a conventional cutpoint of 130), with a relatively high number of false positives and false negatives. The Leiter-R authors point out however, that the error rates in these data may be partially due to error in the criterion variable (gifted identification by local schools), and not simply the error in the Leiter-R.

Similar analyses were performed for children with learning disabilities and those with ADHD. The authors report that the Memory Process Composite and the cognitive/Social Composite scores from the rating scales aid in identifying these individuals. Nonetheless, the overall hit rates for the students with learning disabilities (both Nonverbal and Verbal types) only reached 78% and 76% for the two groups, respectively. The hit rate rates were higher for ADHD and ADD-only groups, 92% and 93%, respectively. In all cases the number of false positives exceeded false negatives to a considerable degree (e.g., 20% to 24% for the students with learning disabilities). The ADD/ADHD and LD data should be evaluated cautiously because of the low number of exceptional children in the samples (e.g., samples ranging from 10 to 20 in size); in addition, all group comparisons are limited because of the failure to include demographically-matched control groups.

In total, data from 11 special groups are reported in the manual. The special groups ranged in size from 3 (Traumatic Brain Injury) to 73 (English as Second Language). FSIQ means for the groups in the 6 to 20 age range and the specific group names are: 83, Severe Speech/Language Impairment; 84, Severe Hearing Impairment; 74, Severe Motor Delay; 77, Traumatic Brain Injury; 55, Cognitive Delay; 89, ADHD/ADD; 115, Gifted; 83, LD-nonverbal; 88, LD verbal; 93, ESL-Spanish; 95, ESL-other). All the mean scores were higher for children in the 2 to 5 year old group, though typically not by much. For example, the ESL-other group was only .2 of one point higher; however, the Speech Impaired groups differed by 8.1 points. Most of the differences were in the 3 to 5 point range. The Memory and Attention scale scores were similar, but in the main, hovered more closely around the population mean of 100. For example, the Memory Screener scores for all ages and all groups ranged from 70 (Cognitive Delay Group) to 111 (Gifted Group).

In summary, the Leither-R is designed to be used primarily for individuals with poor verbal communication skills and/or those from other cultures. The manual provides considerable data to users to aid them in making decisions about the utility of the test for individuals within specific exceptional groups. However, the generalizability of the special group comparison data is suspect due to multiple methodological limitations. Despite some salient limitations, the test exhibits significant strengths. For example, because the test contains 20 subtests, four rating scales, and a variety of scale scores it offers considerable administrative flexibility and offers assessment of a number of constructs. Examiners may find it useful for high stakes decision making.

SUMMARY

The Leiter-R was developed based on a number of current models of intelligence (e.g., the Gf-Gc Model of Cattell, the work of Gustaffson). The normative sample matches the U.S. population fairly well on important stratifying variables and at the total sample level, but the sample-to-population match varies considerably at individual age levels. Although the test is largely nonverbal in its administration, some subtests may require verbalization. Administration directions include an array of gestures and pantomimed instructions that are vast in number and may be confusing. The Leiter-R appears to have adequate reliability at the scale level for an instrument intended for important decision-making (Bracken, 1987, 1988; Nunnally & Bernstein, 1994). Importantly, as a measure of general intelligence the test is composed of subtests that are rated as fair or poor measures of *g*. The instrument matches the proposed four-or-five factor theoretical underpinnings fairly well, with some minor model variation across the age levels. When used with individuals who have recently immigrated to the United States, practitioners should be aware that the Leiter-R contains stimulus materials that are influenced significantly by Western culture.

LEITER-R CASE

The following case is presented to illustrate utility of the Leiter-R. This case was recommended by Gale H. Roid, coauthor of the Leiter-R, and adapted from data originally presented by Armenteros and Roid (1996) during a presentation entitled "Nonverbal Abilities of Hispanic and Speech-Impaired Preschoolers: A Case Study." The case was presented at the Annual Meeting of the American Psychological Association, Toronto, Ontario, Canada.

Psychological Evaluation

Name: John
Age: 3 years, 10 months
Language: English and Spanish

Reason for Referral

John is a 3 year, 10 month old Hispanic male who was referred by his parents for a complete psychoeducational evaluation because of speech and language difficulties, as well as for assistance with educational planning.

Background Information

John is a preschool child of Hispanic descent who has been exposed to both English and Spanish in the household. He lives with his parents, who each have two years of college education, and four older siblings.

The results of a recent speech and language evaluation suggest significant receptive and expressive speech and language deficits in both English and Spanish, including areas of vocabulary and articulation. Mixed language dominance was reported. John's speech intelligibility is reported to be poor to fair, and his spontaneous conversation uses jargon and brief verbal utterances. In addition, John has difficulty responding to open-ended questions.

John's mother reports an uneventful pregnancy. The child was born three weeks prematurely via vaginal delivery, but without complications. Developmental milestones were achieved within normal limits, with the exception of speech and language skills, which were reportedly delayed. John's medical history is unremarkable. He is said to be a healthy child. John's family medical history includes a reading-disabled brother and maternal uncle. John has never attended an educational stimulation program. He has always been cared for by his mother at home. John has not received any previous evaluation or treatment for his speech and language problems.

Socially and behaviorally, John is described as a well-behaved and affectionate child who likes to play with a variety of toys, games, and activities available in the household. He is able to interact adequately with adults, sibling, and other children most of the time. John has certain chores and responsibilities around the house. Verbal reprimands and time-outs are said to be the main disciplinary methods used successfully with John.

Tests Administered

- Sensory Screening
- Leiter International Performance Scale–Revised (Leiter-R)
- Developmental Test of Visual-Motor Integration
- Learning Accomplishment Profile–Diagnostic (LAP-D)
- Scales of Independent Behavior (SIB)
- Conners' Rating Scales (CRS), Parent Scale

Behavioral Observations

John was appropriately dressed and well groomed on the days of the evaluation. He was accompanied by his mother, from whom he separated with ease. He preferentially used his right hand and demonstrated sensory and motor functioning that appeared to be within normal limits.

Communication with John and administration of verbal test items were accomplished bilingually, in English and Spanish, since he has been exposed to both languages. When provided with verbal instructions, John was able to follow simple two-step oral directions, but repetition was usually required. John's speech was characterized by generally poor articulation, and expressive language included jargon and two- to five-word utterances, predominantly in English with some words in Spanish.

Rapport with John was easy to establish as he readily engaged in interaction with the examiner and with the toys and materials provided. He demonstrated appropriate range and intensity of emotions and maintained a friendly and playful attitude during the assessment. John was cooperative and put forth good effort throughout the evaluation process. John's activity level was moderate to excessive, his attention span was short for his age, and his impulse control was fair to poor. He became easily distracted and required frequent structuring and monitoring in order to focus and stay on the task at hand. John's work style was characterized by a combination of trial-and-error and insight in his approach to problem solving. His use of search and scanning skills was below average. John was capable of self-correction and seemed aware of his capabilities and limitations. John generally responded to a combination of positive reinforcement and limit setting.

Test Results

John's test results in cognitive-intellectual, developmental, and functional adaptive behavioral areas are now described.

Cognitive-Intellectual Functioning
On the Leiter International Performance Scale–Revised (Leiter-R), John obtained a Brief IQ of 119, ranking in performance of nonverbal cognitive tasks at the 90th percentile for age and falling within the Above Average range of intellectual ability. The chances are two out of three that his "true score" lies between 114 and 124. The true score is the hypothetical average that would be obtained upon repeated testing, minus the effects of error such as practice and fatigue. Leiter-R items are nonverbal and specifically designed for administration to children with communication disorders, as well as children whose first language is not English.

Results were consistently indicative of above average functioning in most of the nonverbal ability areas assessed, especially in visualization skills, where his highest performance was noted. Reasoning skills were also found to be above average. In contrast, attention and memory skills were somewhat lower, falling within the Average range.

Analysis of John's Leiter-R subtest scores revealed significant strengths in the ability to determine from contextual clues the missing element in a picture and the ability to visually perceive an object or shape embedded in a complex figure. A relative weakness was evident in his ability to perceive a pattern and to hold it in memory long enough to reproduce it several times.

Leiter-R Visualization and Reasoning Battery

Subtest	Scaled Score*
Figure Ground (FG)	16
Form Completion (FC)	13
Matching (M)	12
Sequential Order (SO)	12
Repeated Patterns (RP)	9
Picture Context (PC)	16
Classification (C)	14

Leiter-R Attention and Memory Battery

Subtest	Scaled Score*
Sustained Attention (SA)	11
Forward Memory (FM)	9

* Subtest M = 10, SD = 3.

Developmental Functioning
On the Developmental Test of Visual-Motor Integration (VMI), John obtained an age equivalent score of 3 years, 6 months. His performance on the VMI is therefore generally commensurate with chronological age expectancy level and is indicative of average functioning in visual-perceptual-motor integration skills.

The Learning Accomplishment Profile–Diagnostic (LAP-D) is a standardized test instrument used for the purpose of identifying mastered and emerging developmental achievement skills in preschool and kindergarten children. John obtained the following scores on the eight subscales administered:

LAP-D Subscale	Age Equivalent (months)	Percentile Rank	Standard Score*
Fine Motor: Manipulation	43–44	45	98
Fine Motor: Writing	43–44	46	99
Cognitive: Matching	39–40	35	94
Cognitive: Counting	44–45	50	100
Language: Naming	33–35	3	72
Language: Comprehension	36	11	82
Gross Motor: Body Movement	49–50	85	116
Gross Motor: Object Movement	43–45	54	102

*Subscale M = 100, SD = 15.

Analysis of John's LAP-D profile revealed a significant strength in locomotor skills. On the other hand, significant deficits were evidence in receptive language/comprehension skills and expressive language/naming skills. The standard score that John obtained on the subscale that measures receptive language skills was more than one standard deviation below the chronological age mean, while the standard score obtained on the subscale that assess expressive language skills was almost two standard deviations below expectations.

John's developmental achievement in the following areas was found to be generally age-appropriate and within the Average range: manual dexterity/visuospatial constructional skills, visual-motor integration/pre-writing skills, abstract nonverbal reasoning/perceptual-matching skills, counting skills/quantitative concepts, and object control skills.

The language deficits found in the LAP-D were generally commensurate with the results of the separate bilingual speech and language evaluation, which revealed significant receptive and expressive speech and language deficits in both English and Spanish.

Adaptive Behavioral Functioning

On the Scales of Independent Behavior (SIB), John obtained a Broad Independence Scale standard score of 87 (M = 100, SD = 15) and an age equivalent of 2 years, 9 months, which is suggestive of below-average performance in overall functional independence. A significant weakness was found in communication skills, while average functioning was evident in motor development. These results are generally consistent with the findings of the LAP-D.

The Parent Scale of the Conners' Rating Scales (CRS) was administered in order to assess John's overall behavioral functioning. Based on the ratings provided by John's mother, there were no problem areas reported that were significantly higher than other children of similar age and sex. However, analysis of the individual items endorsed suggests that the following specific concerns were raised: speech is difficult to understand, tends to whine at times, becomes distracted when spoken to, and cries when he does not get his way.

Summary and Recommendations

John is a 3-year-old Hispanic male who is presenting significant speech and language problems in both English and Spanish. Intellectually, he is functioning within the Above Average range of nonverbal cognitive functioning. Developmentally, significant deficits were revealed in both receptive and expressive speech and language skills. These deficits were documented by the results of the LAP-D and the SIB, as well as by the findings of the bilingual speech and language evaluation. John's developmental functioning in the areas of fine motor, gross motor, and cognitive skills, as measured by the LAP-D, and in the area of visual-perceptual-motor skills, as measured by the VMI, was found to be age-appropriate. Behaviorally, below average functioning independence was noted on the SIB, while concerns with inattention and speech and language problems were raised on the CRS.

Based on the results of this evaluation, the following recommendations are made:

1. John would benefit from a preschool program that provides early developmental stimulation in an individual and multimodal format. He should have developmentally age-appropriate experiences in all areas, especially in the areas of speech and language. Educational programming should take into consideration John's average to above average level of nonverbal cognitive functioning.

2. John would benefit from continued exposure to a language-rich environment in which the child's bilingual and bicultural background is considered. The development of speech and language skills should be encouraged at home and in the classroom by promoting supervised social interactions with peers and adults.

3. John would benefit from speech and language therapy.

4. Teachers are recommended to use a positive approach with John, maintaining realistic expectations and praising any improvements.

5. John would benefit from a behavior modification program, both at home and at school, in order to help him attend better and achieve more self-control.

6. John's progress should be closely monitored in order to ensure the ongoing appropriateness of his educational program in meeting his needs. Reevaluation before entering kindergarten is recommended in order to monitor his developmental progress and to better ascertain his future educational needs.

 TEST YOURSELF

I. The age range for the Leiter-R standardization is
(a) 2 years to 20 year, I I months
(b) 2 years to 16 years, I I months
(c) 5 years to 17 years, I I months
(d) 6 years to 17 years, I I months

2. Which subtest yields a g loading greater than .70?
(a) Paper Folding
(b) Matching
(c) Figure Ground
(d) Sustained Attention

3. Which two subtests are included in the Brief IQ Battery?
(a) Figure Ground and Form Completion
(b) Cube Design and Matching
(c) Design Analyses and Classification
(d) Paper Folding and Sustained Attention

4. The subtest with the poorest floor on the AV Battery is

(a) Repeated Patterns

(b) Figure Ground

(c) Form Completion

(d) Figure Rotation

5. In the "Strengths and Weaknesses of Leiter-R Reliability and Validity" section it was indicated that _____ reliabilities are higher than _____ reliabilities.

(a) Split-half : test-retest

(b) Test-retest : split-half

(c) Predictive : test-retest

(d) Predictive : split-half

6. Which of the following was listed as a developmental strength?

(a) Drawings are colorful

(b) Excellent standardization sample for the AM Battery

(c) Development was guided by 10 stated goals

(d) Excellent use of bias panels

7. A limitation of the standardization sample of the Leiter-R is

(a) Overrepresentation of foreign-born children

(b) Atypical weighting

(c) Too many special education children included

(d) Size

8. Of the available nonverbal tests, which one includes four rating scales?

(a) UNIT

(b) CTONI

(c) Leiter-R

(d) GAMA

9. The short form of the Leiter-R requires administration of _____ subtests.

(a) 2

(b) 3

(c) 4

(d) 5

(continued)

10. Of the available nonverbal tests, which test offers the greatest number of subtests?

(a) UNIT

(b) Leiter-R

(c) CTONI

(d) NNAT

Answers: 1. a; 2. a; 3. a; 4. d; 5. a; 6. a.; 7. d; 8. c; 9. c; 10. b

Appendix A

UNIT Interpretive Worksheet

Step 1: Interpret the Full Scale IQ

Scale	IQ	Confidence Interval	Percentile Rank	Descriptive Category
		90/95 Circle one		
Memory		90/95		
Reasoning		90/95		
Symbolic		90/95		
Nonsymbolic		90/95		
Full Scale		90/95		

Note. If there is at least one significant difference between the component parts of the Full Scale IQ (i.e., among the following quotients: Memory [MQ], Reasoning [RQ], Symbolic [SQ], and Nonsymbolic [NSQ]), the Full Scale should not be interpreted as the most meaningful indicator of the individual's overall performance.

Step 2: Are there significant differences among the quotients: Memory, Reasoning, Symbolic, and Nonsymbolic (see Rapid Reference 3.12)?

MQ vs. RQ Difference	Significance	SQ vs. NSQ Difference	Significance
	If yes, circle one		**If yes, circle one**
	.05 .01		.05 .01

If both the answers are no (there are not significant differences between either the MQ and RQ or the SQ and NSQ), first explain the meaning of the scales not being significantly different, then skip to Step 5.

If either answer is yes, there is a significant difference between either the MQ and RQ or the SQ and the NSQ, then continue on to Step 3.

Step 3: Are the MQ vs. RQ or the SQ vs. NSQ differences abnormally large?

Difference	Size needed for Abnormality	Does size meet criteria?	
MQ vs. RQ	20 points (Extreme 15%)	YES	NO
	23 points (Extreme 10%)	YES	NO
	27 points (Extreme 5%)	YES	NO
	34 points (Extreme 1%)	YES	NO
SQ vs. NSQ	20 points (Extreme 15%)	YES	NO
	23 points (Extreme 10%)	YES	NO
	27 points (Extreme 5%)	YES	NO
	34 points (Extreme 1%)	YES	NO

Step 3 Decision Box

If any abnormal differences exist, and if the scatter within any global scale is less than six points, interpret these abnormal differences in Step 4. If no abnormal differences exist, or if excessive scatter exists within one or more global scales, go to Step 5.

Step 4: Interpret the global Memory vs. Reasoning and/or Symbolic vs. NonSymbolic and Nonverbal Differences if they were found to be interpretable (see Table 3.3).

Step 5: Interpret Significant Subtest Strengths and Weaknesses of Profile

A. Determine which mean you should use to calculate strengths and weaknesses.

MQ vs. RQ Discrepancy

0–20 points	Examine SQ vs. NSQ discrepancy
21 or more	Use mean of MQ subtests and RQ subtests separately

B. SQ vs. NSQ

0–20, and MQ vs. RQ < 20	Use mean of all subtests administered (Pooled Procedure)
21 or more	Use mean of SQ subtests and NSQ subtests separately

Subtests	Scaled Score	Rounded Mean	Difference	Strength/Weakness Percentile
Sym mem				
Cube Des				
Spa Mem				
Ana Rea				
Obj Mem				
Mazes				

Appendix B

Leiter-R Interpretive Worksheet

Step 1: Interpret the Full Scale IQ.

Scale	IQ	Confidence Interval	Percentile Rank	Descriptive Category
Brief IQ				
Full Scale IQ				
Fluid Reasoning				
Fundamental Vis				
Spatial Visualization				
Memory Screen				
Associative Memory				
Memory Span				
Attention				
Memory Process				
Recognition Memory				

Note. If there is at least one significant and rare difference between the component parts of the Full Scale IQ (i.e., among the following composites: Fluid Reasoning, Fundamental Visualization, and Spatial Visualization), the Full Scale IQ should not be interpreted as the most meaningful representation of the individual's overall performance.

Step 2: Are there significant differences among the Composites?

Circle, as necessary			
BIQ vs. MS	BIQ vs. MP	FSIQ vs. MS	FSIQ vs. MP
BIQ vs. SV	BIQ vs. FR	BIQ vs. FV	FSIQ vs. SV
FSIQ vs. FR	FSIQ vs. FV	SV vs. FR	FR vs. FV
RM vs. MS	AM vs. Msp	AM vs. MP	AM vs. A
AM vs. MS	Msp vs. MP	Msp vs. A	Msp vs. MS
MP vs. A	MP vs. MS	A vs. MS	

Note. BIQ = Brief IQ Screener; FSIQ = Full Scale IQ; MS = Memory Screener; MP = Memory Process; SV = Spatial Visualization; FR = Fluid Reasoning; FV = Fundamental Visualization; RM = Recognition Memory; AM = Associative Memory; A = Attention; Msp = Memory Span.

If there are no significant differences, explain the meaning of the scales not being significantly different, then skip to Step 5. If there is/are significant difference(s), go on to Step 3.

Step 3: Are the differences abnormally large, that is, larger than the tabled values below?

Circle, as necessary			
BIQ vs. SV	BIQ vs. FR	BIQ vs. FV	FSIQ vs. SV
(18)	(13)	(20)	(13)
FSIQ vs. FR	FSIQ vs. FV	SV vs. FR	FR vs. FV
(16)	(16)	(20)	(26)
RM vs. MS	AM vs. Msp	AM vs. MP	AM vs. A
(20)	(25)	(24)	(26)
AM vs. MS	Msp vs. MP	Msp vs. A	Msp vs. MS
(16)	(12)	(25)	(16)
MP vs. A	MP vs. MS	A vs. MS	
(25)	(16)	(24)	

Note. See Step 2 for explanation of abbreviations.

Step 3 Decision Box

If any abnormal differences exist, and if the scatter within either global scale of a particular comparison is less than nine points, interpret the abnormal differences in Step 4. If no abnormal differences exist, or if excessive scatter exists, go to Step 5.

Step 4: Interpret the composite differences.

Step 5: Interpret significant subtest strengths and weaknesses of subtest profile.

A. Determine which "Rounded Mean" you should use to calculate strengths and weaknesses.

B. Use the following table to determine subtest outliers (strengths and weaknesses), as necessary

Subtests	Score	Rounded Mean					Difference	Strength/ Weakness
		FR	BIQ	FV	FSIQ	SV		
FG								
DA								
FC								
M								
SO								
RP								
PC								
C								
PF								
FR								

Note. FG = Figure Ground; DA = Design Analogies; FC = Form Completion; M = Matching; SO = Sequential Order; RP = Repeated Patterns; PC = Picture Context; C = Classification; PF = Paper Folding; FR = Figure Rotation; FR (of column head) = Fluid Reasoning; BIQ = Brief IQ Screener; FV = Fundamental Visualization; FSIQ = Full Scale IQ; SV = Spatial Visualization.

Subtest	Score	Rounded Mean						Difference	Strength/ Weakness
		MS	AM	Msp	A	MP	RM		
AP									
IR									
FM									
AS									
RM									
VC									
SM									
DP									
DR									
AD									

Note. AP = Associated Pairs; IR = Immediate Recognition; FM = Forward Memory; AS = Attention Sustained; RM = Reverse Memory; VC = Visual Coding; SM = Spatial Memory; DP = Delayed Pairs; DR = Delayed Recognition; AD = Attention Divided; MS = Memory Screener; AM = Associative Memory; Msp = Memory Span; A = Attention; MP = Memory Process; RM (of column head) = Recognition Memory.

References

Armenteros, E. C., & Roid, G. H. (1996, August). *Nonverbal abilities of Hispanic and speech-impaired preschoolers.* Paper presented at the meeting of the American Psychological Association, Toronto, Canada.

Arthur, G. (1925). A new point performance scale. *Journal of Applied Psychology, IX,* 390–416.

Arthur, G. (1943). *A Point Scale of Performance Tests: Clinical Manual.* New York: The Commonwealth Fund.

Arthur, G. (1947). *A Point Scale of Performance Tests: Clinical Manual.* New York: The Commonwealth Fund.

Arthur, G., & Woodrow, H. (1919). An absolute intelligence scale: A study in method. *Journal of Applied Psychology, III,* 118–137.

Bracken, B. A. (1984). *Bracken Basic Concept Scale.* San Antonio, TX: Psychological Corporation.

Bracken, B. A. (1986). Incidence of basic concepts in the directions of five commonly used American tests of intelligence. *School Psychology International, 7,* 1–10.

Bracken, B. A. (1987). Limitations of preschool instruments and standards for minimal levels of technical adequacy. *Journal of Psychoeducational Assessment, 5,* 313–326.

Bracken, B. A. (1988). Ten psychometric reasons why similar tests produce dissimilar results. *Journal of School Psychology, 26,* 155–166.

Bracken, B. A. (1993, October). *Intelligence testing:: Our futures or our past.* Debate with Daniel Reschly conducted at the Michigan Association of School Psychologists' Fall Conference, Shanty Creek, MI.

Bracken, B. A. (1998a). *Bracken Basic Concept Scale–Revised.* San Antonio, TX: Psychological Corporation.

Bracken, B. A. (1998b). *Bracken Basic Concept Scale–Revised: Spanish Form.* San Antonio, TX: Psychological Corporation.

Bracken, B. A., & Fouad, N. (1987). Spanish translation and validation of the Bracken Basic Concept Scale. *School Psychology Review, 16,* 94–102.

Bracken, B. A., & McCallum, R. S. (1998). *Universal Nonverbal Intelligence Test.* Itasca, IL: Riverside.

Bracken, B. A., & McCallum, R. S. (1999). *Universal Nonverbal Intelligence Test: University training guide.* Itasca, IL: Riverside.

Bracken, B. A., Barona, A., Bauermeister, J. J., Howell, K. K., Poggioli, L., & Puente, A. (1990). Multinational validation of the Spanish Bracken Basic Concept Scale for cross-cultural assessment. *Journal of School Psychology, 28,* 325–341.

Braden, J. P. (1999). Straight talk about assessment and diversity: What do we know? *School Psychology Quarterly, 14,* 343–355.

Brown, L., Sherbenou, R. J., & Johnsen, S. K. (1990). *Test of Nonverbal Intelligence* (2nd ed.). Austin: Pro-Ed.

Brown, L., Sherbenou, R. J., & Johnsen, S. K. (1997). *Test of Nonverbal Intelligence* (3rd ed.). Austin: Pro-Ed.

Brown, R. T., Reynolds, C. R., & Whitaker, J. S. (1999). Bias in mental testing since Bias in Mental Testing. *School Psychology Quarterly, 14,* 208–238.

Carpenter, P. A., Just, M. A., & Shell, P. (1990). What one intelligence test measures: A theoretical account of the processing in the Raven's Progressive Matrices Test. *Psychological Review, 97*(3), 404–431.

Carrey, N. J. (1995). Itard's 1828 memoir on "mutism caused by a lesion of the intellectual functions": A historical analysis. *Journal of the American Academy of Child and Adolescent Psychiatry, 341,* 655–1661.

Carroll, J. B. (1993). *Human cognitive abilities: A survey of factor-analytic studies.* New York: Cambridge University Press.

Cattell, R. B. (1963). Theory of fluid and crystallized intelligence. *Journal of Educational Psychology, 54,* 1–22.

Donzelli, J. (1996, September 11). How do you say "milk" in 54 different ways? *Sun Sentinel* (Fort Lauderdale), East Broward Edition, Community Closeup section, p. 11.

Dunn, L. M., & Dunn, L. M. (1981). *Peabody Picture Vocabulary Test–Revised.* Circle Pines, MN: American Guidance Service.

Elliott, C. D. (1990). *Differential Ability Scales: Administration and scoring manual.* San Antonio, TX: The Psychological Corporation.

Fachting, A., & Bradley-Johnson, S. (in press). A review of the Universal Nonverbal Intelligence Test (UNIT). *Psychology in the Schools.*

Fast Fact. (1996, December 5). *Sun Sentinel* (Fort Lauderdale), Palm Beach Edition, Local section, p. 1B.

Fives, C., & Flanagan, R. (2000). *A review of the Universal Nonverbal Intelligence Test (UNIT): An advance for evaluating youth with diverse needs.* Manuscript submitted for publication.

Forester, S. (2000, March 13). *Personal Communication.*

Frijda, N., & Jahoda, G. (1966). On the scope and methods of cross-cultural research. *International Journal of Psychology, 1,* 109–127.

Frisby, C. L. (1999). Straight talk about cognitive assessment and diversity. *School Psychology Quarterly, 14,* 195–207.

Gittler, G., & Tanzer, N. K. (1998). *Establishing cross-cultural equivalence of item complexity using the linear logistic test model (LLTM).* Paper presented at the Symposium on Cross-Cultural Assessment and Test Adaptations 24th International Congress of Applied Psychology, San Francisco.

Glutting, J. J., McDermott, P. A., & Konold, T. R. (1997). Ontology, structure, and diagnostic benefits of a normative subtest taxonomy from the WISC-III standardization sample. In D. P. Flanagan, J. L. Genshaft, & P. L. Harrison (Eds.), *Contemporary intellectual assessment: Theories, tests, and issues* (pp. 349–372). New York: Guilford.

Government Printing Office. (1918). *Examiners Guide for Psychological Examining in the Army.* Washington, DC: Author.

Gulliksen, H. (1987). *Theory of mental tests.* Hillsdale, NJ: Erlbaum. (Original work published 1950)

Gustaffsson, J. E. (1984). A unifying model for the structure of intellectual abilities. *Intelligence, 8,* 179–203.

Hammill, D. D., Pearson, N. A., & Wiederholt, J. L. (1996). *Comprehensive Test of Nonverbal Intelligence.* Austin, TX: Pro-Ed.

Harcourt Brace Educational Measurement. (1996). *Stanford Achievement Test, Ninth Edition.* San Antonio, TX: Author.

Harcourt Brace Educational Measurement. (1997). *Aprenda: La prueba de logros en Espanol, segunda edicion.* San Antonio, TX: Author.

Healy, W. L. (1914). A Pictorial Completion Test. *The Psychological Review,* 189–203.

Healy, W. L. (1918). *Pictorial Completion Test II.* Chicago: C. H. Stoelting.

Healy, W. L. (1921). Pictorial Completion Test II. *Journal of Applied Psychology, 5,* 232–233.

Hilliard, A. G., III (1984). IQ testing as the emperor's new clothes: A critique of Jensen's Bias in Mental Testing. In C. R. Reynolds & R. T. Brown (Eds.), *Perspectives on bias in mental testing* (pp. 139–169). New York: Plenum.

Horn, J. L. (1968). Organization of abilities and the development of intelligence. *Psychological Review, 75,* 242–259.

Horn, J. L., & Cattell, R. B. (1966). Refinement and test of the theory of fluid and crystallized general intelligences. *Journal of Educational Psychology, 57*(5), 253–270.

Hunter, J. E., & Hunter, R. F. (1984). Validity and utility of alternative predictors of job performance. *Psychological Bulletin, 96*(1), 72–98.

Individuals with Disabilities Education Act. (1997). (IDEA, 20 U.S.C. 1400 et seq.)

Itard, J. M. G. (1932). *The wild boy of Aveyron.* New York: Appleton-Century-Crofts.

Jensen, A. R. (1980). *Bias in mental testing.* New York: Free Press.

Kaufman, A. S. (1979). *Intelligent testing with the WISC-R.* New York: Wiley.

Kaufman, A. S. (1990). *Assessing adolescent and adult intelligence.* Boston: Allyn & Bacon.

Kaufman, A. S. (1994). *Intelligent testing with the WISC-III.* New York: Wiley.

Kaufman, A. S., & Kaufman, N. L. (1983). *Interpretive manual for the Kaufman Assessment Battery for Children (K-ABC).* Circle Pines, MN: American Guidance Service.

Kaufman, A. S., & Kaufman, N. L. (1983). *Kaufman Assessment Battery for Children: Administration and scoring manual.* Circle Pines, MN: American Guidance Service.

Kaufman, A. S., & Kaufman, N. L. (1990). *Kaufman Brief Intelligence Test Manual.* Circle Pines, MN: American Guidance Service.

Kaufman, A. S., & Lichtenberger, E. O. (1999). *Essentials of WAIS-III Assessment.* New York: Wiley.

Kellogg, C. E., & Morton, N. W. (1934). Revised Beta Examination. *Personnel Journal, 13,* 98–99.

Kellogg, C. E., & Morton, N. W. (1999). *Beta III Manual.* San Antonio, TX: Psychological Corporation.

Knox, H. A. (1914). A scale based on the work at Ellis Island for estimating mental defect. *Journal of the American Medical Association, 62,* 741–747.

Kohs, S. C. (1919). *Intelligence measurement.* New York: Macmillan.

Kohs, S. C. (1919). *Kohs Block Design Test.* Wood Dale, IL: Stoelting.

Leiter, R. G. (1979). *Instruction Manual for the Leiter International Performance Scale.* Wood Dale, IL: Stoelting.

Lindner, R. M., & Gurvitz, M. (1946). Restandardization of the Revised Beta Examination to yield Wechsler type of IQ. *Journal of Applied Psychology, 30,* 649–658.

Lipman, H. (1997, August 3). A change in ethnic demographics presents new challenges, opportunities. *The Times Union,* p. A1.

Lonner, W. J. (1985). Issues in testing and assessment in cross-cultural counseling. *The Counseling Psychologist, 13,* 599–614.

Maller, S. J. (1999). *The Universal Nonverbal Intelligence Test: A promising instrument for assessing deaf children.* Paper presented at the annual meeting of the National Association of School Psychologists, Las Vegas.

McCallum, R. S. (1991). The assessment of preschool children with the Stanford-Binet Intelligence Scale–Fourth edition. In B. A. Bracken (Ed.), *The pychoeducational asessment of peschool children* (2nd ed., pp. 107–132). Boston: Allyn & Bacon.

McCallum, R. S. (1999). A "baker's dozen" criteria for evaluating fairness in nonverbal testing. *School Psychologist, 40*–60.

McCallum, R. S., & Bracken, B. A. (1999). *Fairness issues in cross-cultural assessment: The Universal Nonverbal Intelligence Test.* Invited paper presented at the Joint Conference of the International Association for Cross-Cultural Psychology and the International Test Commission.

McDermott, P. A., Fantuzzo, J. W., & Glutting, J. J. (1990). Just say no to subtest analysis: A critique on Wechsler theory and practice. *Journal of Psychoeducational Assessment, 8,* 290–302.

McDermott, P. A., & Glutting, J. J. (1997). Informing stylistic learning behavior, disposition, and achievement through ability subtests—Or, more illusions of meaning? *School Psychology Review, 26,* 163–175.

McGrew, K. S. (1994). *Clinical interpretation of the Woodcock-Johnson tests of cognitive ability–Revised.* Boston: Allyn & Bacon.

McGrew, K. S., & Flanagan, D. P. (1998). *The intelligence test desk reference (ITDR): Gf-Gc cross-battery assessment.* Boston: Allyn & Bacon.

Montgomery, J. W., Windsor, J., & Stark, R. E. (1991). Specific speech and language disorders. In J. E. Obrzut & G. W. Hynd (Eds.), *Neuropsychological foundations of learning disabilities: A handbook of issues, methods, and practice* (pp. 573–601). San Diego, CA: Academic.

Naglieri, J. A. (1985a). *Matrix Analogies Test–Expanded Form.* San Antonio, TX: Psychological Corporation.

Naglieri, J. A. (1985b). *Matrix Analogies Test–Short Form.* San Antonio, TX: Psychological Corporation.

Naglieri, J. A. (1985). Use of the WISC-R and K-ABC with learning disabled, borderline mentally retarded, and normal children. *School Psychology Review, 22,* 133–141.

Naglieri, J. A. (1996). *Naglieri Nonverbal Ability Test.* San Antonio, TX: Psychological Corporation.

Naglieri, J. A. (1996). *NNAT multilevel technical manual.* San Antonio. TX: Harcourt Brace Educational Measurement.

Naglieri, J. A. (1997). *Naglieri Nonverbal Ability Test 3/4 multilevel form technical manual.* San Antonio, TX: Harcourt Brace Educational Measurement.

Naglieri, J. A., & Bardos, A. N. (1997). *General Ability Measure for Adults.* Minneapolis, MN: NCS Assessments.

Naglieri, J. A., & Kaufman, A. S. (1983). How many factors underlie the WAIS-R? *Journal of Psychoeducational Assessment, 1,* 113–119.

Naglieri, J. A., & Ronning, M. E. (in press). *Comparison of White, African American, Hispanic, and Asian Children on the Naglieri Nonverbal Ability Test.* Manuscript submitted for publication.

Nunnally, J., & Bernstein, I. H. (1994). *Psychometric theory (3rd Edition).* New York: Mc-Graw-Hill.

O'Hanlon, A. (1997, May 11). Non-English speakers are testing schools. *The Washington Post,* Prince William Extra section, p. V01.

Pasko, J. R. (1994). Chicago—Don't miss it. *Communique, 23*(4), 2.

Pinter, R., & Patterson, D. G. (1917). *A scale of performance tests.* New York: Appleton.

Porteus, S. D. (1915). Mental tests for the feebleminded: A new series. *Journal of Psycho-Asthenics, 19,* 200–213.

Power, S. (1996, May 9). Panel suggests school clerks learn Spanish: Board takes no action on report. *The Dallas Morning News,* Plano section, p. 1F.

Prifitera, A., & Saklofske, D. (1998). *WISC-III: Clinical use and interpretation.* New York: Academic.

Prifitera, A., Weiss, L. G., & Saklofske, D. H. (1998). The WISC-III in context. In A. Prifitera & D. H. Saklofske (Eds.), *WISC-III clinical use and interpretation: Scientist-practitioner perspectives* (pp. 1–38). New York: Academic.

Puente, M. (1998, May 27). Californians likely to end bilingual ed. *USA Today,* News section, p. 4A.

Raven, J. C. (1960). *Guide to using the standard progressive matrices.* London: H. K. Lewis.

Raven, J., Raven, J. C., & Court, J. H. (1998). *Manual for Raven's Progressive Matrices and Vocabulary Scales.* Oxford, UK: Oxford Psychologists Press.

Reynolds, C. R., Lowe, P. A., & Saenz, A. L. (1999). The problem of bias in psychological assessment. In C. R. Reynolds & T. B. Gutkin (Eds.), *Handbook of school psychology* (3rd ed., pp. 549–595).

Roid, G. H., & Miller, L. J. (1997). Leiter International Performance Scale–Revised: Examiner's manual. In G. H. Roid & L. J. Miller (Eds.)., *Leiter International Performance Scale–Revised.* Wood Dale, IL: Stoelting.

Rourke, B. P. (Ed.). (1995). *Syndrome of nonverbal learning disabilities: Neurodevelopmental manifestations.* New York: Guilford.

Saccuzzo, D. P., & Johnson, N. E. (1995). Traditional psychometric tests and proportionate representation: An intervention and program evaluation study. *Psychological Assessment, 7*(2), 183–194.

Sattler, J. M. (1988). *Assessment of children* (3rd ed.). San Diego, CA: Author.

Sattler, J. M. (1992). *Assessment of children* (3rd ed. rev.). San Diego, CA: Author.

Savich, P. A. (1984). Anticipatory imagery ability in normal and language-disabled children. *Journal of Speech and Hearing Research, 27*(4), 494–501.

Searcey, D. (1998, February 9). Tukwila high school is true cultural melting pot. *The Seattle Times,* South section, p. B1.

Seguin, E. (1907). *Idiocy and its treatment by the physiological method.* New York: Teachers College, Columbia University.

Spearman, C. (1927). *The abilities of man: Their nature and measurement.* New York: Macmillan.

Steele, M. (1998, January 23). Bilingual education program an expensive failure. *The Arizona Republic,* Northeast Phoenix Community section, p.2.

Stepp, D. (1997, November 20). School watch; as demographics change, language programs grow; transition help: the international welcome center helps non-English-speaking students adjust. *The Atlanta Journal and Constitution,* Extra section, p. 02g.

Sternberg, R. J., & Powell, J. S. (1982). Theories of intelligence. In R. J. Sternberg (Ed.), *Handbook of human intelligence* (pp. 975–1006). New York: Cambridge University Press.

Styles, I., & Andrich, D. (1993). Linking the standard and advanced forms of the Raven's Progressive Matricies in both the pencil-and-paper and computer-adaptive-testing formats. *Educational & Psychological Measurement, 53*(4), 905–925.

Thorndike, R. M., & Lohman, D. F. (1990). *A century of ability testing.* Chicago: Riverside.

Thorndike, R. L., Hagen, E. P., & Sattler, J. M. (1986). *Stanford-Binet Intelligence Scale–Fourth Edition technical manual.* Itasca, IL: Riverside.

U.S. Bureau of the Census. (1995). *Current population survey, March 1995.* Washington, DC: Author.

U.S. Department of Education. (1995). *Seventeenth annual report to congress on the implementation of the Individuals with Disabilities Education Act.* Washington, DC: Author.

Ulik, C. (1997, January 6). Civil rights officials check Tempe schools; limited-English programs studied. *The Arizona Republic/The Phoenix Gazette,* Tempe Community Section, p.1.

Unz, R. (1997, October 19). Perspective on education; bilingual is a damaging myth; a system that ensures failure is kept alive by the flow of federal dollars. A 1998 initiative would bring change. *Los Angeles Times,* Opinion section, part M, p.5.

Van Duch, M. (1997, January 19). Learning that other language—English—can be fun. *Chicago Tribune,* Tempo Northwest section, Zone: NW, p. 2.

Wasserman, J. D, Becker, K. A., McCallum, R. S., & Bracken, B. A. (2000). *Toward a methodology for Universal Norming Adaptation for nonverbal tests.* (Unpublished manuscript).

Wechsler, D. (1939). *Measurement of adult intelligence.* Baltimore: Williams and Wilkins.

Wechsler, D. (1944, 1955, 1981). *Manual for the Wechsler Adult Intelligence Scale.* San Antonio, TX: Psychological Corporation.

Wechsler, D. (1949). *Wechsler Intelligence Scale for Children.* San Antonio, TX: Psychological Corporation.

Wechsler, D. (1991). *Wechsler Intelligence Scale for Children–Third edition.* San Antonio, TX: Psychological Corporation.

Wechsler, D. (1992). *Wechsler Individual Achievement Test.* San Antonio, TX: Psychological Corporation.

Woodcock, R. W. (1990). Theoretical foundations of the WJ-R measures of cognitive ability. *Journal of Psychoeducational Assessment, 8,* 231–258.

Woodcock, R. W., & Johnson, M. B. (1989/1990). *Woodcock-Johnson Psycho-Educational Battery–Revised.* Itasca, IL: Riverside.

Yerkes, R. M. (Ed.). (1921). *Memoirs of the National Academy of Sciences: Vol. 15. Psychological examining in the United States Army.* Washington, DC: U.S. Government Printing Office.

Yoakum, C. S., & Yerkes, R. M. (1920). *Army Mental Tests.* New York: Holt.

Annotated Bibliography

AERA, APA, & NCME. (1999). *Standards for educational and psychological testing.* Washington, DC: AERA.

As suggested by the title, this document provides standards for test developers and consumers.

Bracken, B. A. (1987). Limitations of preschool instruments and standards for minimal levels of technical adequacy. *Journal of Psychoeducational Assessment, 5,* 313–326.

This article provides guidelines for psychometric standards for preschool ability tests. These standards have been fairly widely adopted by test publishers and have been applied to ability tests serving populations of all ages. Instruments reviewed in the current book are compared to the standards described in this article.

Bracken, B. A., & McCallum, R. S. (1998). *Universal Nonverbal Intelligence Test.* Itasca, IL: Riverside.

The UNIT is one of two current and comprehensive nonverbal tests of intelligence. The UNIT Examiner's Manual presents many advances in the assessment of intelligence and psychometric applications (e.g., local reliabilities, chapter dedicated to fairness in testing).

Bracken, B. A., Barona, A., Bauermeister, J. J., Howell, K. K., Poggioli, L., & Puente, A. (1990). Multinational validation of the Spanish Bracken Basic Concept Scale for cross-cultural assessment. *Journal of School Psychology, 28,* 325–341.

This article illustrates state-of-the-art procedures for test translation and validation. Using the Bracken Basic Concept Scale as the vehicle for translation, the validity of the multinational, multidialectical translation of the BBCS was assessed in Puerto Rico, Venezuela, and the southwestern United States.

Braden, J. (Ed). (in press). Major nonverbal measures of intelligence and special abilities: Special monograph issue.

Special issue of the Journal of Psychoeducational Assessment, *devoted entirely to empirical studies and reviews. All articles focus on major nonverbal tests of intelligence and special abilities including the UNIT, Leiter-R, and others.*

Brown, L., Sherbenou, R. J., & Johnsen, S. K. (1997). *Test of nonverbal intelligence* (3rd ed.). Austin: Pro-Ed.

The TONI-III is a widely used unidimensional test of intelligence. The Manual provides a brief history of testing and the theoretical rationale for the test, as well as administration, scoring, and interpretation guidelines.

Carrey, N. J. (1995). Itard's 1828 memoir on "mutism caused by a lesion of the intellectual functions": A historical analysis. *Journal of the American Academy of Child and Adolescent Psychiatry, 341,* 655–1661.

Carrey's article describes an historical case in which traditional language-oriented approaches to assessment proved less than beneficial. Itard's challenge was to assess the intelligence of and provide meaningful intervention for the "Wild Boy of Aveyron." This historical precedent sets the stage for professional efforts to assess and address the needs of children with language-related differences or disabilities.

Fachting, A., & Bradley-Johnson, S. (in press). Review of Universal Nonverbal Intelligence Test. *Psychology in the schools.*

This review describes the theoretical background and primary test characteristics of the UNIT, including reliability, validity, fairness, and some of the administration, scoring, and interpretative features. The review is generally positive in tone.

Flannagan, R., & Five, C. (2000). *Review of Universal Nonverbal Intelligence Test: An advance for evaluating youths with diverse needs.* St. John's University: Review submitted for publication.

This test review offers a description of the UNIT's theoretical background and primary test characteristics (including a critical review of reliability, validity, and fairness), and some comments on administration, scoring, and interpretation. The review provides a good treatment of strengths and weaknesses of the test, and is generally positive.

Flynn, J. R. (1999). Searching for justice: The discovery of IQ gains over time. *American Psychologist, 54*(1) 5–20.

Flynn presents a summary of findings commonly known as the "Flynn Effect," which illustrates that on average the population is gaining in assessed intelligence at a rate of about three IQ points per decade. Flynn addresses potential reasons for this phenomenon.

Government Printing Office. (1918). *Examiner's guide for psychological examining in the army.* Washington, DC: Author.

This publication provides readers with an interesting historical perspective and insight into the development of the Army Alpha and Beta Batteries. Most notable about this publication is the discernable lineage of instruments as they have progressed from the early test developers to today's current authors' batteries.

Hammill, D. D., Pearson, N. A., & Wiederholt, J. L. (1996). *Comprehensive Test of Nonverbal Intelligence.* Austin, TX: Pro-Ed.

This test provides a matrix analogies format for assessing intelligence. The Manual *provides a definition of nonverbal intelligence, a brief history of nonverbal assessment, and a description of the CTONI, including the rationale and administration, scoring, and interpretation guidelines.*

Jensen, A. R. (1980). *Bias in mental testing.* New York: Free Press.

Jensen's book is considered by many to be the preeminent treatise on detecting test bias, and on various other issues related to bias in mental testing.

Naglieri, J. A. (1996). *Naglieri Nonverbal Ability Test.* San Antonio, TX: Psychological Corporation.

This is a group-administered test of intelligence. The Manual describes the rationale for the test, a strong standardization sample, and other relevant technical, administration, scoring, and interpretation features. As is the case with many group-administered tests, it is used often for screening purposes.

Naglieri, J. A., & Bardos, A. N. (1997). *General Ability Measure for Adults.* Minneapolis, MN: NCS Assessments.

This is a group-administered test of intelligence designed for adults. It is used often as a screening device.

Raven, J. C. (1960). *Guide to using the Standard Progressive Matrices.* London: H. K. Lewis.

This guide provides the administrative and scoring information necessary to use the Standard Progressive Matrices Test.

Roid, G. H., & Miller, L. J. (1997). *Leiter International Performance Scale–Revised.* Wood Dale, IL: Stoelting.

The Leiter International Performance Scale was once the standard for assessing children with limited language facility or disability. The original Leiter fell from favor when its norms and test materials became too dated. Roid and Miller accepted the task of revising and renorming the venerable Leiter, and they completed the task successfully in 1997.

Sattler, J. M. (1992). *Assessment of children* (3rd ed. rev.). San Diego, CA: Author.

Sattler provides relatively comprehensive coverage of major tests of intelligence and special abilities, including a section on the background and history of several nonverbal measures. The book also covers many relevant assessment issues, including history and models of intelligence testing, relevant theories of intelligence, attention to the nature/nurture issue, and so forth, as well as the theoretical background of instruments, test/subtest descriptions, and some details of administration, scoring, and interpretation.

Thorndike, R. M., & Lohman, D. F. (1990). *A century of ability testing.* Chicago: Riverside.

Thorndike and Lohman provide a concise and thorough description of efforts to define and assess the construct of intelligence through a variety of means, including nonverbal procedures.

Index

About the Authors

R. Steve McCallum is Head of the Department of Educational Psychology at the University of Tennessee. He was trained as a School Psychologist at the University of Georgia, and worked full-time for about four years in applied settings. Since 1986 he has been a trainer of school psychologists; he served as Director of the School Psychology Program at the University of Tennessee before becoming Department Head in 1988. He still engages in the delivery of applied services as a supervisor of students in the schools, as a consultant to local schools, and through his work in a private practice setting. He is the author of over 100 scholarly works, including articles, national and international conference presentations, and book chapters. In addition, he is cofounder and co-editor of the *Journal of Psychoeducational Assessment* and coauthor of the Universal Nonverbal Intelligence Test (UNIT). Dr. McCallum was elected as a Fellow of APA's Division 16 in 1992.

Bruce A. Bracken obtained his PhD at the University of Georgia in 1979. Currently, he is a Professor of School Psychology at The College of William & Mary. During his career, Dr. Bracken has authored more than 100 articles, reviews, chapters, books, curricula, and tests related to psychological constructs and psychoeducational assessment. Among his major publications are the *Bracken Basic Concept Scale–Revised,* the *Bracken Concept Development Program,* the *Multidimensional Self Concept Scale,* the *Assessment of Interpersonal Relations,* and the *Universal Nonverbal Intelligence Test,* which he co-authored with R. Steve McCallum. His previous books include edited texts, the *Psychoeducational Assessment of Preschool Children,* and the *Handbook of Self-Concept.* He cofounded and co-edits the *Journal of Psychoeducational Assessment,* and he sits on several national and international journal boards. He is a Fellow in the American Psychological Association and a Diplomate of the American Board of Psychological Assessment. Dr. Bracken currently is President Elect of the International Test Commission and is a former Chair of the APA Committee on Psychological Testing and Assessment.

John D. Wasserman, PhD, is a clinical neuropsychologist and test developer. While serving as the Director of Psychological Assessments at Riverside Publishing, Itasca, Illinois, he directed development of the revision of the *Stanford-Binet Intelligence Scale* and the *Bender Visual Motor Gestalt Test.* He has previously directed the development of the *Das-Naglieri Cognitive Assessment Sys-*

tem (CAS) and the *Universal Nonverbal Intelligence Test* (UNIT). Prior to joining Riverside Publishing, he worked as a project director for The Psychological Corporation, where he directed such projects as the *Devereux Behavior Rating Scales; NEPSY: A Developmental Neuropsychological Assessment;* revisions of the *California Verbal Learning Test;* the *Delis-Kaplan Executive Function Scales;* and the behavior rating scale from the *Bayley Scales of Infant Development–Second Edition.* In 1999, he served as Chair of the Clinical Division of the Association of Test Publishers. Dr. Wasserman has taught graduate courses in personality and psychopathology, psychological assessment, neuropsychology, and statistics and research methods. He is presently an Adjunct Associate Professor in Educational Psychology at the University of Tennessee, Knoxville. He has also taught at several other universities, including Trinity University, San Antonio; Loyola University, New Orleans; and the University of Miami, Coral Gables, Florida. The author of over 50 papers and professional presentations, Dr. Wasserman is a licensed psychologist and directed a pediatric neuropsychology service at Children's Hospital in New Orleans before becoming a test developer. He obtained his PhD in 1990 in clinical psychology from the University of Miami and completed a two-year fellowship in clinical neuropsychology at L.S.U. and Tulane University Medical Centers from 1987–1989.